Case

Studies

in

Medicine

CASE STUDIES IN MEDICINE

K L Gupta MB, MRCP
Associate Professor
Department of Medicine
New York Medical College

WITH A FOREWORD BY

Richard D Levere MD
Professor and Chairman
Department of Medicine
New York Medical College, and
Director, Department of Medicine
University Hospital/Wetchester
County Medical Center

CHURCHILL LIVINGSTONE
EDINBURGH LONDON MELBOURNE AND NEW YORK 1986

CHURCHILL LIVINGSTONE
Medical Division of Longman Group UK Limited

Distributed in the United States of America by Churchill Livingstone Inc., 1560 Broadway, New York, N.Y. 10036, and by associated companies, branches and representatives throughout the world.

First published 1986
Reprinted 1989

ISBN 0-443-03633-0

Produced by Longman Singapore Publishers (Pte) Ltd
Printed in Singapore

IN MEMORY OF
MY FATHER AND UNCLE

FOREWORD

This book represents Dr Krishan Lal Gupta's third published contribution towards the preparation of candidates for the MRCP. His first, *100 Short Cases for the MRCP*, was written while Dr. Gupta was Senior Registrar in Geriatric Medicine at London Hospital. That book has become almost required reading for candidates taking the MRCP and has been published in translation, allowing its more extensive use in other countries. His second book, *Multiple Choice Questions in Geriatric Medicine*, is already widely used by students preparing for the multiple choice questions format used in the MRCP and similar examinations. This present book is Dr Gupta's first since coming to the United States and, although it is intended for candidates for the MRCP, it appears to have relevance also for those taking not only the American Board of Internal Medicine, but for students of U.S. and Canadian medical schools who are preparing for the National Board examination in Internal Medicine.

The author's professed goal is to provide the student with a mechanism for thinking about common medical problems utilizing a problem-solving approach to diagnosis. The 100 case presentations all represent the type of medical problems that frequently present to the practitioner and all require the student to use his or her 'data base' of pathophysiologic information in a rational, logical and cost-effective way in order to come to a specific diagnostic impression. The physician must learn to think in such a manner, rather than to memorize unconnected pieces of data, so that he or she is equipped to handle the rapidly changing scientific and technological base of medicine. I like to compare this with utilizing the 'rifle' rather than the 'shotgun' approach to clinical diagnosis. These is no doubt that this method of teaching will be most useful to physicians sitting for the MRCP but will prove, in addition, to be extremely helpful to students studying Internal Medicine in all countries, including the U.S., because of Dr Gupta's use of a problem-solving approach to clinical diagnosis.

New York, 1986 — Richard D. Levere M.D.

PREFACE

The art of arriving at a meaningful conclusion from history, physical signs and initial, albeit limited, investigations is essential for the practice of good quality medicine. In recent years increasing awareness of cost containment in patient care has made it much more important that students of medicine acquire the skills of synthesizing the acquired information into the most likely diagnosis and plan for the most appropriate investigations and management. Most medical textbooks are good enough for giving detailed accounts of the multitude of diseases, but only few teach the students how to process the available data into the most probable diagnosis. This technique of problem solving in medicine, of course, requires constant practice and rational thinking.

This book discusses 100 medical problems as they commonly (at times with atypical features) present to the practising physician in a typical district general hospital. All of these cases comprise genuine clinical problems and are not simply 'grey' cases. The book aims precisely to give students of medicine a chance to practise and improve their skill in problem solving. Not only qualifying students (final MB, MRCP, MRCGP and equivalent examinations in various other countries) but almost all practising physicians should find the case studies an interesting, challenging and stimulating exercise.

K Gupta, MB, MRCP

CASE 1

A lady of 75 was admitted with a 1-hour history of sudden severe chest pain radiating to her lower jaw, with shortness of breath. She was sent to the medical ward after being given parenteral frusemide and diamorphine in the casualty department.

On examination she was found to be dyspnoeic and had central cyanosis. JVP was raised by 4 cm but she had no ankle oedema, clubbing or lymphadenopathy. She had triple rhythm and was fibrillating with an apical rate of 160/min. She had diffuse bilateral basal crepitations with occasional rhonchi. Examination of abdomen and central nervous system was normal.

Over the next 2 hours her chest pain settled but she was still in fast fibrillation with a rate of about 150/min. The houseman at this stage gave her a dose of 1 mg of digoxin parenterally and prescribed a further 0.25 mg twice a day for the next 48 hours. After 24 hours she was reported to have difficulty in differentiating red from green and blue, and also complained of nausea and sickness. Her pulse rate at this stage was 78/min irregular.

The results of various investigations were as follows:

Haemoglobin 12.4 g/dl
ESR 33 mm/h
Sodium 136 mmol/l
Potassium 3.4 mmol/l
Chloride 97 mmol/l
Bicarbonate 24 mmol/l
WBC 6.8 × 10^9/l
Blood glucose 7.4 mmol/l
Blood urea 12 mmol/l
Chest X-ray – Heart size enlarged; bilateral pulmonary congestion
Urine analysis normal

Questions

1 What is the most likely diagnosis?
2 How would you confirm your diagnosis?
3 Name four other drugs that may cause changes in colour vision?
4 Name three other drugs which may be used for atrial fibrillation.

Answers to case 1

1 The most likely diagnosis in this elderly lady is digoxin toxicity. Apart from the gastrointestinal symptoms (nausea and vomiting) and various cardiac dysrhythmias, digoxin may cause colour vision changes (red, green and blue defects), especially in the elderly.

2 Serum digoxin level if over 2.5 ng/ml would indicate digoxin toxicity.

3 (a) Barbiturates
(b) Quinine and chloroquine
(c) Antiepileptic drugs such as tridione
(d) Antitubercular drugs such as isoniazid

4 (a) Quinidine
(b) Verapamil
(c) Amiodarone

CASE 2

A man of 47 was admitted with a 4-hour history of central chest pain and shortness of breath. His pain radiated to the left shoulder and lower jaw and was moderate to severe in intensity. He was diagnosed to have angina 3 months ago and was advised to lose weight and take glyceryl trinitrate tablets as required. He had tried three tablets before coming into the hospital but with no benefit. He had taken a sumptuous meal the night before and since he thought the pain might have been due to indigestion he had also tried some milk of magnesia but this did not help the pain either. He had felt nauseated in the last 2 hours and had perspired a lot. He had been fit and healthy until 3 months ago. He lived with his wife and had two sons, 18 and 16 years old. He had smoked 25 cigarettes a day for over 25 years until 3 months ago when he stopped smoking on his doctor's advice. His father died at the age of 53, his mother was 68 and healthy and one brother, 51, was also in good health.

On examination he was obese; JVP was not raised. Blood pressure was 130/70. Pulse was 68/min with occasional extrasystole. Respiration was 20/min. There was no cyanosis, thyroid enlargement or lymphadenopathy. His heart was in sinus rhythm with occasional extrasystole, but heart sounds were normal. He had a soft systolic apical murmur with no radiation. Trachea was central, breath sounds were normal with few left basal crepitations. Examination of abdomen and central nervous system proved normal.

The results of various investigations were as follows:

Haemoglobin 14.9 g/dl
WBC 9.7 × 10^9/l
Sodium 140 mmol/l
Potassium 3.5 mmol/l
Chloride 99 mmol/l
Bicarbonate 23 mmol/l
Urea 8.4 mmol/l
Random blood glucose 8 mmol/l
ECG – changes of inferior myocardial infarction seen
Chest X-ray – Heart size normal; normal lung fields
Urine analysis normal

The condition improved after treatment with morphine, oxygen and bed rest, and he was allowed to sit out on the third day of his admission. However, on the same evening he suddenly became dyspnoeic and complained of tightness in his chest. His blood pressure dropped to 90/50, pulse was 40/min and respiratory rate was 34/min. On examination at this stage he was found to have developed a pansystolic apical murmur radiating to the left axilla. There was no evidence of deep vein thrombosis in the legs. His chest was full of basal crepitations bilaterally. Examination of central nervous system and abdomen remained unremarkable.

Questions

1 What is the most likely cause of this patient's deterioration on the third day of his admission?
2 How should papillary muscle rupture be treated?
3 Name six complications of myocardial infarction which may be seen within the first week.

Answers to case 2

1 ***Initial diagnosis in this 47-year-old obese gentleman, with history of smoking and family history of heart disease with recently diagnosed angina with acute onset of chest pain radiating to left shoulder and lower jaw, is myocardial infarction. This diagnosis was of course confirmed on the ECG. Papillary muscle rupture is not an uncommon complication in the first week and typically presents with signs of shock and left ventricular failure. The sudden appearance of pansystolic apical murmur, falling blood pressure, pulmonary congestion and tachypnoea are also suggestive of this complication in this patient.***

2 ***Papillary muscle rupture requires immediate assessment and treatment with***
(a) Morphine
(b) Oxygen
(c) Digoxin
(d) Dopamine to increase the blood pressure
(e) Consideration of surgical intervention in cases of failure of medical therapy.

3 ***(a) Various cardiac arrhythmias***
(b) Congestive cardiac failure
(c) Cardiogenic shock
(d) Pericarditis
(e) Rupture of interventricular septum, chordae tendinae, or the myocardium
(f) Thromboembolism

CASE 3

A man of 53 was admitted with chronic obstructive airways disease, hypertension, ischaemic heart disease and congestive cardiac failure. His heart failure was controlled with digoxin and increasing dose of frusemide. Four days after his admission he complained of painful swelling of his right knee. He denied any history of trauma.

On examination at this stage he was plethoric but not dyspnoeic. His raised JVP and oedema of legs had subsided with the treatment he had received during the first 4 days. His blood pressure was 180/100, his pulse was 84/min and regular, and there was no clubbing or lymphadenopathy. His apex beat was in the fifth intercostal space about 1 cm outside the midclavicular line. He had no murmurs. In the respiratory system he had a few basal crepitations and scattered rhonchi. Abdomen and central nervous system were normal. He had moderate effusion of his right knee with painful limitation of movements. Examinations of other joints was normal. His haemoglobin was reported as 18 g/dl and an X-ray of his right knee was reported as showing changes of osteo-arthritis with no bony injury.

Other investigation results were as follows:

Blood urea 11 mmol/l
Blood sugar 6.4 mmol/l
Total protein 67 g/l
Albumin 32 gm/l
Bilirubin 14 μmol/l
Sodium 130 mmol/l
Potassium 3.2 mmol/l
Chloride 97 mmol/l
Bicarbonate 27 mmol/l
Chest X-ray (on arrival) – Emphysematous lungs with bilateral pulmonary congestion and some blunting of the right costophrenic angle; heart size enlarged

Questions

1 What is the most likely diagnosis, and why?
2 Name four drugs which may precipitate an acute gouty attack.
3 Name three haematological disorders which may cause secondary gout?
4 What is the single most helpful investigation for differentiating gout from pseudogout?

Answers to case 3

1 The most likely diagnosis is an acute gouty attack affecting his right knee precipitated by massive doses of diuretics. His haemoglobin of 18 g/dl is indicative of secondary polycythaemia associated with chronic obstructive airways disease. Polycythaemia is a well-known cause for secondary gout. Although the first metatarsophalangeal joint is usually involved, gout may affect any joint and may, in fact, occur in more than one joint at a time.

2 (a) Diuretics such as thiazide and frusemide
(b) Low-dose salicylates
(c) Cytotoxic drugs
(d) Antituberculous drugs such as pyrazinamide and ethambutol

3 (a) ***Polycythaemia***
(b) ***Leukaemia***
(c) ***Haemolytic anaemia***

4 ***Aspiration of the joint is the most helpful investigation in differentiating gout from pseudogout. In gout the characteristic needle-shaped crystals of sodium biurate are seen under the microscope, whereas in pseudogout the crystals are of calcium pyrophosphate dihydrate and have a different shape.***

CASE 4

A 72-year-old man was admitted after a mild left-sided stroke and recovered with little residual weakness within 2 weeks. His blood pressure was 150/90 and his pulse was 82/min regular. There were no significant abnormalities on examination apart from the signs of upper motor neurone hemiparesis affecting his left side. Routine urine examination was normal. He was independent enough to be discharged to his own home.

A day before discharge he mentioned his failing vision which he thought had been gradually coming on for over 3 months. An outpatient appointment was arranged in 3 weeks time in the ophthalmology department for his eye trouble. When seen he was noted to be walking with a stick; there was no evidence of visual field defect. He had a small lenticular opacity in his left eye. Intraocular pressure, light and accommodation reflexes and eye movements were noted to be normal on both sides. Discs were normal too, but there were hard exudates on the temporal side with microaneurysms in both eyes. He could count the fingers with both eyes tested separately.

The following were the results of various investigations:

Haemoglobin 13.4 g/dl
ESR 42 mm/h
WBC 9×10^9/l
Sodium 139 mmol/l
Potassium 4.0 mmol/l
Chloride 100 mmol/l
Bicarbonate 24 mmol/l
Blood glucose 9.2 mmol/l (fasting)
Blood urea 7.3 mmol/l
Urine analysis normal
Chest X-ray – No cardiomegaly; lung fields clear, ECG – Sinus rhythm, some T wave inversion in left chest leads (V_{3-6})

Questions

1 What is the cause for this man's failing vision?
2 How do you explain the absence of glycosuria in the urine on his recent admission?
3 What is the treatment of his retinopathy?
4 Give four important causes of gradual loss of vision in old age.

Answers to case 4

1 Probably diabetic retinopathy and lenticular opacity of his left eye.

2 Because of the increased renal threshold the diagnosis of diabetes may be missed in up to 50 per cent of the elderly diabetics on simple routine urine examination. A fasting blood sugar therefore is much more appropriate in elderly subjects.

3 (a) Adequate control of his diabetes
(b) Laser treatment for his retinopathy

4 (a) Senile cataract
(b) Chronic glaucoma
(c) Senile macular degeneration
(d) Retinopathy (diabetic/hypertensive)

CASE 5

A 48-year-old lady was referred by her doctor for further investigation, with moderate splenomegaly for no obvious cause. She admitted experiencing excessive tiredness, lethargy and general weakness for the past 4 months but this, she thought, was because of pressure of work. She had been given a course of ampicillin 6 weeks ago for her cough and cold. She denied any history of serious illness in the past.

She lived alone in a second-floor council flat and worked as a part-time secretary in a local store. She did not smoke or drink, and strongly believed that both were bad for health. Her only sister who lived in Scotland had myxoedema.

On examination she was not anaemic. There was no oedema, clubbing or lymphadenopathy. JVP not raised. She was mildly jaundiced but there were no spider naevi or palmar erythema. Her liver was 2 cm enlarged, smooth and non-tender. The spleen was 4 cm enlarged. There was no ascites. Respiratory, cardiovascular and central nervous systems were normal. She had osteoarthritis of both knees but could walk unaided. Blood results were as follows:

Haemoglobin 13 g/dl
ESR 46 mm/h
Sodium 139 mmol/l
Potassium 3.4 mmol/l
Chloride 99 mmol/l
Urea 7 mmol/l
Blood sugar 11 mmol/l
MCV 89 fl
WBC 8 × 10^9/l
Bilirubin 47 μmol/l
Protein 63 g/l
Albumin 27 g/l
AST 190 μ/l
Alkaline phosphatase 150 u/l

Questions

1 What is the differential diagnosis?
2 What three further investigations will favour the diagnosis of chronic active hepatitis?
3 Name two more investigations that you consider are relevant
4 Give four conditions known to be associated with chronic active hepatitis

Answers to case 5

1 The differential diagnosis in this lady with general ill health, hepatosplenomegaly, jaundice, raised serum enzymes and bilirubin, low serum albumin and high globulin is chronic hepatitis or cirrhosis (cryptogenic).

2 (a) Liver biopsy (lymphocytic or plasma cell infiltration)
(b) Serum immunoglobulin assay (IgG in excess of 2 g/dl)
(c) Persistent elevation of hepatic enzymes

3 (a) Australia antigen (B surface antigen, e antigen and antibody)
(b) Alpha fetoprotein
(c) Autoantibodies, e.g. antinuclear, smooth muscle and antimitochondrial antibodies

4 (a) Ulcerative colitis
(b) Hashimoto's disease
(c) Thyrotoxicosis
(d) Glomerulonephritis

CASE 6

A 69-year-old retired schoolteacher was admitted with 2 month history of painful ulcers on the tips of her fingers, heartburn and progressive shortness of breath on exertion. She reported that her fingers had been going pale and bloodless in cold weather.

On examination she was mildly anaemic. On her fingertips she had lesions of telangiectasia and small vasculitic ulcers. Skin over the fingers and dorsum of both hands was taut and thickened with areas of hypopigmentation. Skin around the mouth was smooth and waxy. Blood pressure was 160/88, pulse 80/min regular. JVP was not raised. Lymphadenopathy nil. No clubbing or thyroid enlargement. Cardiovascular, abdomen and central nervous system examination proved normal. Trachea was central. Chest expansion was poor with bilateral fine basal crepitations but adequate air entry.

The following investigation results were available:

Haemoglobin 10.8 g/dl
MCV 89 fl
ESR 45 mm/1st hour
Bilirubin 12 μmol/l
Sodium 142 mmol/l
Potassium 4.1 mmol/l
Chloride 100 mmol/l
Blood sugar 6.7 mmol/l
ECG normal
Protein 69 g/l
Albumin 39 g/l
AST 18 u/l
Alkaline phosphatase 73 u/l

Questions

1 What is the most likely diagnosis?
2 What six investigations will help the diagnosis?
3 What is the treatment of scleroderma?

Answers to case 6

1 The most likely diagnosis in this elderly lady with Raynaud's phenomenon, heartburn (gastrointestinal tract involvement) and dyspnoea (lung involvement), thick and taut skin with vasculitis is scleroderma.

2 (a) X-ray of hands
(b) Chest X-ray
(c) Lung function tests (reduced pulmonary diffusing capacity)
(d) Barium meal and follow-through
(e) Antinuclear antibodies
(f) Skin biopsy

3 Unfortunately no specific therapy is available as yet. Reflux oesophagitis may be helped by antacids and H_2 antagonists such as cimetidine. Steroids are not of much help in the treatment but may be indicated in this patient with progressive pulmonary involvement. Intra-arterial reserpine has been found helpful for Raynaud's phenomenon.

CASE 7

A 36-year-old housewife presented with a 3-month history of excessive weight gain, facial hair growth and weakness. She had gained about 9 pounds in weight during the past 3 months. Her diet and level of physical activities had not changed significantly. She had found the facial hair growth embarrassing and in spite of the fact that she had shaved frequently she had not felt like going out in recent weeks. She felt generally depressed and weak. There was no history of urinary symptoms and her bowels were normal. She lived with her husband and three young children. Her periods were regular and she was not taking any drugs (including pills). She was a non-smoker and drank only occasionally. There was no significant of past illness.

On examination she was obese, weight was 157 lb, height 5 ft 1 in. JVP was normal. Blood pressure was 160/100. Pulse was 78/min regular. Peripheral pulses were normal. There was no anaemia, cyanosis, jaundice, clubbing or oedema. She had a few hairs on her chin. Examination of respiratory system and abdomen proved normal. Her fundi were normal and she had no neurological abnormalities.

Results of the following investigations were available:

Haemoglobin 13.8 g/dl
MCV 91 fl
WBC 6.8 × 10^9/l
Sodium 150 mmol/l
Potassium 3.2 mmol/l
Chloride 101 mmol/l
Bicarbonate 24 mmol/l
Chest X-ray – Heart size normal; no active lung lesion seen
ECG – normal

Questions

1 What is the most likely diagnosis?
2 What are the causes of Cushing's syndrome?
3 What further five investigations will help your diagnosis?

Answers to case 7

1 The most likely diagnosis in this lady with obesity, weight gain, excessive hair growth, weakness, mildly raised blood pressure, high serum sodium and low serum potassium is Cushing's syndrome.

2 (a) Excessive secretion of ACTH by the pituitary gland
(b) Hyperfunction of adrenal cortex (adenoma/carcinoma)
(c) Exogenous administration of steroids

3 (a) Measurement of morning and evening plasma cortisol levels. High levels of plasma cortisol with loss of diurnal variation will suggest the diagnosis
(b) Measurement of free cortisol in the urine. High urinary output of free cortisol would be expected
(c) Dexamethasone suppression test. Small-dose dexamethasone test is done to establish that the patient has hypercortisolism, whereas a large-dose dexamethasone test is used to determine whether the adrenal function is under pituitary control or not. In cases of excessive ACTH secretion from the pituitary, the suppression of adrenal function is seen. Patients with adrenal tumour and ectopic ACTH syndrome fail to show significant suppression. Measurements of ACTH level help in such circumstances as ACTH is low in autonomous adrenal function but is raised in ectopic ACTH syndrome
(d) Chest X-ray and X-ray of the pituitary fossa
(e) Abdominal CT scan

CASE 8

A man of 67, a retired accountant, was admitted with a history of confusion and forgetfulness for the past 6 weeks. For the past 5 days he had been experiencing increasing weakness of his left side and had at least two falls. There was no history of headaches, blurring of vision or loss of consciousness. He lived alone and had smoked 20 cigarettes a day for many years.

On examination his speech was normal, he was pleasantly confused and thought that he was staying in a hotel. He could remember his home address only with great difficulty. There were signs of left-sided upper motor neurone seventh nerve palsy with left-sided hemiparesis with an upgoing plantar on the same side. There was some suggestion of early clubbing of fingers but examination of respiratory and cardiovascular systems was completely normal.

Chest X-ray was reported as showing a right hilar mass with normal lung fields and no cardiac enlargement.

Over the next week his left-sided weakness progressed, he became bedridden, developed bronchopneumonia and died.

Questions

1 What is the most likely diagnosis?
2 What two further investigations would have been helpful in this patient?
3 How often do patients with brain tumours present with epilepsy?
4 How do you differentiate the confusional state caused by brain tumour from senile dementia?

Answers to case 8

1 Carcinoma of the bronchus with brain secondaries is the most likely diagnosis in this patient. Brain tumours, either primary or secondary metastatic deposit, are not uncommon in the fifth and sixth decade and may present diagnostic difficulties because of the atypical clinical presentation and similarities with cerebrovascular disease.

2 (a) Sputum for malignant cells
(b) CT brain scan to confirm a space-occupying lesion

3 Less than 10 per cent of the patients with brain tumours present with an epileptic fit. In other words, only a small percentage of elderly patients with epilepsy have brain tumours. Aetiology of epilepsy in most cases in non-neoplastic.

4 Senile dementia is usually characterized by slowly progressing loss of memory, intellect and personality. A rapid onset and deterioration over a period of weeks, rather than months and years, and the presence of focal signs, is against the diagnosis of senile dementia.

CASE 9 A 53-year-old man with late-onset diabetes was admitted with painful right thigh and difficulty in climbing the stairs for the past 2 weeks. He had been taking chlorpropramide 250 mg daily for the past 17 years. Recently he had experienced excessive thirst and polyurea, and had lost half a stone in weight over the past 3 weeks. He had attended the casualty department following a fall while getting out of the bath about 10 days ago but was sent home since there was no evidence of bony injury on the X-rays of his pelvis and hips.

On examination he was mentally alert. There was no clubbing, lymphadenopathy, anaemia or oedema. Examination of respiratory and cardiovascular systems and abdomen proved normal. He had hard exudates in his fundi, bilateral wasting of thigh muscles but there were no sensory changes. Reflexes were normal apart from sluggish knee-jerks on both sides.

Results of investigations were as follows:

Haemoglobin 14 g/dl
Haemoglobin A_{1c} 30%
ESR 32 mm/1st hour
MCV 87 fl
WBC 10×10^9/l
Blood sugar (random) 23 mmol/l
Urea 13 mmol/l
Potassium 5.2 mmol/l
Sodium 140 mmol/l
Chloride 100 mmol/l
Bicarbonate 21 mmol/l
Urine – sugar +++; no ketones

Questions

1 What is the most likely diagnosis?
2 Give two investigations which will help the diagnosis?
3 What is the significance of blood results of HbA_{1c} of 30 per cent?
4 Give two measures helpful in treating this patient.

Answers to case 9

1 This 53-year-old gentleman with diabetes and retinopathy probably has diabetic amyotrophy as suggested by his proximal muscular weakness and painful thighs, with no sensory deficit. It seems that his diabetes has been out of control recently, as is the case in most patients with diabetic amyotrophy.

2 (a) Electromyography
(b) Muscle biopsy

3 The level of haemoglobin A_{1C} is used as a cumulative index of general level of hyperglycaemia in diabetic patients: if over 10 per cent it represents a poor control of diabetes. It takes a few weeks for the haemoglobin A_{1c} to fall once good control has been re-established.

4 (a) Good control of diabetes mellitus
(b) Physiotherapy

CASE 10

A man of 69 was admitted via the accident and emergency department to the medical unit with coma. History from the wife suggested that he had been generally unwell for the past fortnight, had been forgetful at times and was also getting progressively short of breath on exertion. The wife had noted that her husband had experienced swelling of both his legs for the past two months. He had been frequently taking aspirin tablets for his headaches but preferred not to bother his doctor and had been to the surgery only once about 12 years ago.

Further history from the wife revealed that the patient had retired to bed about 8 o'clock in the evening and after an hour was found by his wife to be having fits.

On examination he was found to be unrousable but responded to painful stimuli. His blood pressure was 210/140, pulse 80/min regular, JVP was raised by 4 cm and there was pitting oedema of both legs. There was no neck stiffness. The fundi showed papilloedema, arteriovenous nipping, flame-shaped haemorrhages and soft exudates on both sides. There were no definite localizing signs but his left plantar was upgoing with generalized hyperreflexia. Apex beat was in the sixth intercostal space about 2 cm outside the midclavicular line, and there was a pansystolic murmur over the apex radiating to the left axilla. Lung bases were full of crepitations but the air entry was not impaired.

Results of various investigations were as follows:

Haemoglobin 12.4 g/dl
WBC 8 × 10^9/l
Total protein 58 g/l
Albumin 29 g/l
Sodium 140 mmol/l
Potassium 3.3 mmol/l
Bicarbonate 24 mmol/l
Chloride 100 mmol/l
Blood urea 14 mmol/l
Blood glucose 10 mmol/l

Questions

1 What is the most likely diagnosis, and why?
2 What three investigations would you ask for?
3 What are the three important aspects of his immediate therapy?

Answers to case 10

1 Malignant hypertension (high blood pressure with papilloedema) with signs of stroke and a grand mal fit all point towards a diagnosis of hypertensive encephalopathy in this patient. Subarachnoid haemorrhage is another possibility but the absence of neck stiffness and subhyaloid haemorrhages make it less likely. Cerebral haemorrhage is usually associated with more marked focal neurological signs.

2 (a) Blood urea and electrolytes
(b) Urine examination for protein, cells and casts
(c) X-ray of the chest

3 (a) To gently control his blood pressure by hydralazine or diazoxide
(b) To treat the heart failure by parenteral loop diuretics such as frusemide
(c) To use dexamethasone to reduce the cerebral oedema

CASE 11

A man of 70 was admitted with history of frequent falls and poor mobility for the past 2 months. His son, who visited him about twice a week, reported that because of his father's frequent falls he had recently arranged a downstairs bed for him. However, this had not helped matters as his father had had three further falls over the weekend and had to be admitted as an emergency. There was no history of associated convulsions or loss of consciousness.

On examination he was found to be mentally alert, his blood pressure was 170/100, pulse 76/min regular. JVP was normal and there was no oedema, lymphadenopathy or carotid bruit. He had rather a staring look with infrequent blinking and poor expression on his face and had a soft and quiet voice. His chest and cardiovascular systems were normal. He was noted to have some tremor of his right thumb and fingers at rest. The tone was somewhat increased in all his limbs but the reflexes were normal.

The following were the results of various investigations:

Haemoglobin 13.1 g/dl
ESR 38 mm/1st hour
Sodium 144 mmol/l
Potassium 4.3 mmol/l
Chloride 101 mmol/l
Bicarbonate 23 mmol/l
Blood urea 4.2 mmol/l
Blood glucose 7.8 mmol/l
Chest X-ray – Normal heart size; no lung lesion seen

Questions

1 What is the most likely diagnosis?
2 What are the three other causes of Parkinsonism?
3 What is the most widely used drug for Parkinsonism?
4 What are the common side effects of levodopa therapy?

Answers to case 11

1 Clinical manifestations such as tremor at rest, rigidity and poverty of movements, expressionless face and soft quiet voice all favour a diagnosis of Parkinsonism. The diagnosis is not always easy, especially in the early stages when the clinical features may not be marked.

2 (a) Drugs such as phenothiazine
(b) Postencephalitic Parkinsonism
(c) Arteriosclerotic Parkinsonism

3 Levodopa

4 (a) Nausea and vomiting
(b) Confusion, depression, hallucinations
(c) Worsening of tremors
(d) Postural hypotension

CASE 12

Mrs B. L., a 63-year-old lady was admitted via the accident and emergency department with a sudden history of collapse with loss of consciousness for 3 hours. History from the husband revealed that she complained of sudden severe left frontal headache and simply fell on the floor just after getting out of his car. She also had an attack of vomiting consisting of a small quantity of clear fluid.

In the past history she had never been ill enough to be in hospital, but the husband could remember that his wife was told 3 years ago by her GP that she had high blood pressure, and was asked to take some tablets regularly. She took these tablets whenever she could remember.

On examination she was found to be deeply comatosed. Her blood pressure was 220/130, pulse 68/min regular, JVP was not raised, there was no lymphadenopathy. In the cardiovascular system she had an ejection systolic murmur at the apex radiating to the right side of her neck. Her chest was clear and there were no abdominal findings. She had marked neck stiffness, left-sided ptosis and the left pupil was somewhat bigger and slower to react to light. She had a flaccid paralysis of her right side. On fundus examination she was found to have marked bilateral arteriovenous nipping but there was no evidence of papilloedema. Reflexes were brisk on the right side with an upgoing plantar.

The following were the results of various investigations:

Haemoglobin 11.9 g/dl
ESR 30 mm/1st hour
MCV 92 fl
Sodium 140 mmol/l
Potassium 3.4 mmol/l
Chloride 100 mmol/l
Bicarbonate 26 mmol/l
Blood urea 13 mmol/l
Blood glucose 10 mmol/l
Chest X-ray – Heart size moderately enlarged; no active lung lesion seen

Questions

1 What is your most likely diagnosis, and why?
2 How do you explain her ptosis?
3 What is the prognosis of this patient?
4 Name two most important investigations for this patient.

Answers to case 12

1 The most likely diagnosis in this lady is subarachnoid haemorrhage. History of previous hypertension, sudden onset of symptoms with headache and finding of neck stiffness and rapid deterioration in consciousness all suggest this diagnosis.

2 Probably an aneurysm at the junction of the posterior communicating artery and posterior cerebral artery pressing on the third nerve nucleus is the explanation for ptosis in this patient.

3 The prognosis in most patients of subarachnoid haemorrhage presenting with coma is very poor.

4 (a) Lumbar puncture.
(b) Carotid angiography.

CASE 13

L. C., a 79-year-old man, was admitted with 2 month history of poor general health, tiredness and bruising over his lower limbs. There was no history of cough, expectoration, chest pain or palpitation. His appetite had not changed recently but he admitted that he was never a big eater. He denied any history of loss of weight. He had not been taking any drugs. He lived alone in a council flat and had hardly any visitors. His only daughter was in Canada. Because of his stubborn nature he refused to accept help from the social services and turned away the meals-on-wheels after just a week, 6 months ago. His diet consisted of coffee, bread and tinned food. He took hardly any fresh fruits or vegetables.

On examination he was anaemic, apathetic and edentulous. Blood pressure was 140/70, pulse 88/min regular, JVP not raised. No clubbing, thyroid or glandular enlargement. He had extensive perifollicular haemorrhages over his thighs and buttocks. Petechial haemorrhages and purpuric spots were also noted on both legs and feet. Examination of cardiovascular, respiratory, abdomen and neurological systems was unremarkable.

The following were the results of various investigations:

Haemoglobin 10.2 g/dl
MCV 89 fl
ESR 24 mm/1st hour
Urea and electrolytes normal
Chest X-ray normal
WBC 8 × 10^9/l
Platelet count normal
Prothrombin time normal
Urine examination normal

Questions

1 What is the most likely diagnosis?
2 Give two investigations which will help the diagnosis.
3 Give five complications of scurvy.

Answers to case 13

1 The most likely diagnosis in this elderly man (living on his own on a diet devoid of fresh fruit and vegetables) with anaemia, perifollicular and petechial haemorrhages on his thighs and legs with normal platelet count and prothrombin time, is scurvy.

2 (a) Estimation of leukocytic ascorbic acid level
(b) Estimation of urinary excretion after a 'loading' dose of vitamin C

3 (a) Extensive haemorrhages and haemarthrosis
(b) Slow wound healing
(c) Delayed or non-union of fractures
(d) Accelerated osteoporosis
(e) Sudden death

CASE 14

A 66-year-old lady was admitted with an 18-month history of dyspepsia, heartburn and regurgitation made worse by lying flat at night and occasional difficulty in swallowing solid foods only. Her doctor diagnosed her as having hiatus hernia with reflux oesophagitis and she responded adequately with magnesium trisilicate and probanthine. Over the past 4 weeks her symptoms suddenly worsened and she started having increasing difficulty not only with solids but liquids as well, with frequent vomiting containing small quantities of undigested food. She had lost her appetite and was in fact scared of eating anything. She lost 1 stone in weight over this period. She could sometimes feel the food sticking behind her sternum.

On examination she looked pale and emaciated. There was no thyroid or lymph node enlargement. Her throat appeared normal. Blood pressure 140/80, pulse 84/min regular. Skin was normal. There was no clubbing, cyanosis or jaundice. Abdominal examination was normal; in particular there was no epigastric mass or tenderness. The rest of the systemic examination was normal too.

The following were the results of various investigations:

Haemoglobin 8.9 g/dl
ESR 47 mm/h
Sodium 138 mmol/l
Chloride 96 mmol/l
Bicarbonate 29 mmol/l
Blood glucose 6.4 mmol/l
WBC 10 × 10^9/l
Chest X-ray – No lung lesion; heart size normal
ECG normal except some flattening of T-wave in left chest leads (V_{3-6})
Barium meal – Stricture at lower end of oesophagus

Questions

1 What could be the final diagnosis?
2 Give five other causes of dysphagia.

Answers to case 14

1 The elderly lady has rather a long history of dyspepsia, heartburn, regurgitation and dysphagia which is characteristic of reflux oesophagitis and hiatus hernia. Her symptoms were only partially relieved with antacid and probanthine, and have in fact become more continuous and persistent during the last 4 weeks. Weight loss and worsening symptoms with the finding of oesophageal stricture on barium meal are certainly suggestive of carcinoma of lower end of oesophagus, and endoscopy and histological confirmation of the lesion is mandatory in this case. There is, however, no strong evidence of benign strictures changing into malignancy.

2 (a) Pseudobulbar palsy
(b) Systemic sclerosis
(c) Achalasia cardia
(d) Oesophageal web (Plummer Vinson/Kelly Patterson syndrome)
(e) Sjögren syndrome

CASE 15

A 29-year-old schoolteacher presented with a 6-week history of weight loss, painful ankles, weakness, undue fatigue and difficulty in keeping with daily routine. She had been in her present job for the past 4 years, had a 6-year old son and had been living happily with her husband who was an accountant working locally. Her appetite had not been so good and she had lost about 8 pounds of weight during the past 6 weeks. There was no history of chest pain, cough, expectoration or palpitation. She had experienced some stiffness in both hands and excessive redness over her cheeks in the past 10 days. She had no previous illnesses apart from occasional migraine-type headaches which she had suffered for over 10 years. She was a keep-fit fanatic and took regular yoga exercises. Three years ago she had become a vegetarian.

On examination her blood pressure was 135/80. Pulse was 88/min regular. Temperature was 37°C. She had no anaemia, jaundice, thyroid or lymph node enlargement. She had an erythematous rash over her face covering both cheeks and the centre of her nose. Joints of hands and ankles appeared to be somewhat puffy but their movements were satisfactory and painless. Her chest was clear. Heart sounds were normal with no murmur. Spleen was 2 cm enlarged and non-tender. Liver was not palpable and there was no ascites. Neurological examination was completely normal.

The following were the results of various investigations:

Haemoglobin 11.9 g/dl
MCV 82 fl
WBC 8.8 × 10^9/l
Polymorphs 69%
Lymphocytes 27%
Eososinophils 3%
Total serum proteins 45 g/l
Albumin 30 g/l
Serum bilirubin 12 μmol/l
Sodium 136 mmol/l
Potassium 3.9 mmol/l
Chloride 100 mmol/l
Bicarbonate 24 mmol/l
Urea 8.9 mmol/l
Chest X-ray – Heart size normal; no active lung lesion seen
ECG normal
Urine analysis – Protein ++; hyaline and granular cast +; RBC 4–6/HPF; WBC 2–4/HPF

Questions

1 What is the most likely diagnosis?
2 What three further investigations will help your diagnosis?
3 Give three drugs which may be used to treat SLE.

Answers to case 15

1 The most likely diagnosis in this young schoolteacher with history of weight loss, arthralgia, fatigue, weakness, skin lesion over her face (butterfly rash), renal involvement and splenomegaly is systemic lupus erythematosus (SLE). The clinical features of SLE

have a wide variability in different patients. The American Rheumatism Association recommendations suggest a minimum of four of the following features: facial erythema; discoid lupus; Raynaud's phenomenon; alopecia; photosensitivity; oral or naso-pharyngeal ulceration; arthritis without deformity; LE cells; chronic false-positive STS; proteinuria over 3.5 g in 24 hours; cellular casts; pleuritis, pericarditis or both; psychosis, convulsions or both; haemolytic anaemia, leucopenia, thrombocytopenia or any combination of the three.

2 (a) ESR
(b) Anti-DNA antibody
(c) Serum complement estimation

3 (a) Steroids
(b) Azathioprine
(c) Chloroquine

CASE 16

A 72-year-old lady was taken to her doctor by her caring daughter, with 3 month history of general ill-health, tiredness, swelling of legs and occasional confusion. Her doctor found her pale and in mild heart failure, and arranged for haemoglobin and other blood tests. Her haemoglobin was found to be 5.6 g/dl and she was admitted to the hospital at the request of her doctor for further investigations and treatment. She denied having abdominal pain but did admit to occasional indigestion and belching. There was no history of loss of appetite or weight, urinary or bowel symptoms. She enjoyed her regular meals-on-wheels, and was visited by a home help once a week and her daughter almost daily.

On examination she was anaemic and mildly confused. Blood pressure was 130/70, pulse 88/min regular, and she had pitting oedema over both ankles. JVP was raised by 2 cm. There was no clubbing, cyanosis, thyroid or lymphadenopathy. Her liver was 3 cm, enlarged, soft, smooth and tender. There was no epigastric mass or tenderness and no splenomegaly or ascites. She had a few bilateral basal crepitations. She was in sinus rhythm and had a soft systolic murmur at the apex. There were no localizing neurological signs.

The following were the results of various investigations:

Haemoglobin (repeated) 5.6 g/dl
WBC 7.8 × 10^9/l
MLV 64 fl
ESR 42 mm/1st hour
Urea 11.3 mmol/l
Potassium 3.6 mmol/l
Chloride 97 mmol/l
Bicarbonate 24 mmol/l
Two stools for occult blood were positive
Chest X-ray – Heart size slightly enlarged; some pulmonary congestion
Barium enema normal

Questions

1 What is the most likely diagnosis?
2 What two further investigations can help the diagnosis?
3 Give three complications of peptic ulcer.

Answers to case 16

1 The most likely diagnosis in this elderly lady with general ill-health, very low haemoglobin with low MCV, and a normal barium enema with positive faecal occult blood is gastric carcinoma or peptic ulcer. Peptic ulcer in old age may be completely asymptomatic or may present only with vague epigastric discomfort and 'indigestion'. This patient also has a mild heart failure, probably as a result of severe anaemia.

2 (a) Barium meal.
(b) Upper gastrointestinal endoscopy.

3 (a) Haemorrhage.
(b) Perforation.
(c) Obstruction.

CASE 17

A man of 38 presented with a 4-month history of increasing weakness, tiredness and fatigue. His appetite had not been so good lately and he had lost 8 pounds in weight over the past 4 months. His bowel habits had remained normal and there were no urinary symptoms. He denied having any cough, expectoration, dyspepsia, chest pain, palpitation, headaches or blurring of vision. He worked as a foreman and lived with his wife and two young children in a terraced house. He had smoked 10 cigarettes a day for the past 15 years but did not drink.

On examination he had an asthenic build. Blood pressure was 110/60. Pulse was 80/min regular. He appeared to be pale but there was no jaundice, cyanosis, clubbing or oedema. JVP was normal and all the peripheral pulses were palpable. There was some brown discolouration of the mucus surface of his lips and buccal mucosa. Teeth and gums were normal. Examination of respiratory and cardiovascular systems, abdomen and central nervous system proved normal.

The following were the results of various investigations:

Haemoglobin 11.6 g/dl
MCV 84 fl
WBC 8 × 10^9/l
ESR 27 mm/h
Sodium 134 mmol/l
Potassium 5.1 mmol/l
Chloride 99 mmol/l
Bicarbonate 24 mmol/l
Urea 3.9 mmol/l
Blood glucose (random) 4.1 mmol/l
Chest X-ray – Heart size normal; no active lung lesion seen
ECG normal
Urine analysis normal

Questions

1 What is the most likely diagnosis?
2 Give three other causes of buccal pigmentation.
3 What four further investigations will help your diagnosis?
4 Give four important causes of Addison's disease

Answers to case 17

1 The most likely diagnosis in this 38-year-old gentleman with weakness, tiredness, fatigue, weight loss, asthenic build, lowish blood pressure, pallor, buccal pigmentation, lowish serum sodium and high potassium, is Addison's disease.

2 (a) Peutz–Jeghers syndrome
(b) Arsenic, bismuth or silver intake
(c) Metastatic malignant melanoma

3 (a) Plain X-ray abdomen
(b) Adrenal antibodies
(c) Synacthen test
(d) Mantoux test

4 (a) Idiopathic atrophy (the commonest)
(b) Infection (tuberculous and fungal)
(c) Infiltration (metastasis, amyloidosis)
(d) Acute adrenal haemorrhage (Waterhouse Friedrichsen syndrome)

CASE 18

L.C., a 66-year-old retired sales manager, was admitted with cough, dyspnoea on exertion and wheezing, particularly in the morning for the past 3 weeks. His symptoms had started with a cold for the first 3 days. He had little mucoid phlegm. He had tried a cough mixture without much help. There was no history of chest pain, palpitation or haemoptysis. His appetite and bowels had been normal and he denied any history of weight loss. He lived with his wife and had never smoked. He had recently been under stress since his only son had been charged by the police in connection with a burglary.

On examination he was not anaemic. There was no clubbing or lymphadenopathy. Blood pressure 140/90, pulse 80/min regular, thyroid not enlarged, no cyanosis. JVP was not raised. Trachea was central, chest expansion was poor on both sides with bilateral scattered rhonchi and few basal crepitations. Cardiovascular, abdomen and neurological systems were normal.

Initial investigation results were as follows:

Haemoglobin 13.9 g/dl
WBC 8 × 10^9/l
ESR 40 mm/1st hour
Sodium 139 mmol/l
Potassium 3.5 mmol/l
Chloride 100 mmol/l
Bicarbonate 26 mmol/l
Blood urea 10.9 mmol/l
Blood glucose 7 mmol/l
Urine analysis normal
ECG – Sinus rhythm; occasional ventricular ectopics

Questions

1 What is the most likely diagnosis?
2 What four investigations will you ask for?
3 Name one collagen disease which may present with bronchial asthma.

Answers to case 18

1 The most likely diagnosis in this 66-year-old non-smoker gentleman with unproductive cough, dyspnoea on exertion, wheeziness with widespread rhonchi all over his chest and normal ECG is late-onset bronchial asthma. Asthma may appear for the first time in middle age or later.

2 (a) Absolute eosinophil count
(b) Chest X-ray
(c) Lung function test (vitallograph before and after bronchodilator to demonstrate reversible airways obstruction)
(d) Sputum for eosinophils

3 Polyarteritis nodosa

CASE 19

A man of 59, a retired accountant, was admitted with 6 month history of increasing tiredness and lethargy and 2 month history of poor appetite. He had gained half a stone in weight over the past 6 weeks. There was no history of cough, expectoration, chest pain or palpitation. His bowel habits had remained unchanged. He was started on frusemide 3 weeks ago by his GP but this had not helped matters and in fact had worsened his tiredness. He had enjoyed 2 pints of beer a day and 15 cigarettes a day for the past 15 years. For the past 3 weeks he had been almost housebound.

On examination he was mentally alert and was clinically mildly icteric with bilateral pitting oedema of legs. JVP was normal and there was no clubbing or lymphadenopathy. He had marked spider naevi on his left face and upper chest and bilateral palmar erythema with an early Dupuytren's contracture on his left palm. Respiratory and cardiovascular systems were normal. He had significant fluid thrill and shifting dullness in his abdomen with some venous dilatation over his abdominal wall. There was no venous hum. His liver was not palpable but the spleen was moderately enlarged. There were no significant neurological signs.

Initial blood results were repeated:

Haemoglobin 11.4 g/dl
MCV 93 fl
ESR 49 mm/h
WBC 6.7 × 10^9/l
Urea 4.2 mmol/l
Sodium 136 mmol/l
Potassium 2.9 mmol/l
Total protein 70 g/l
Serum albumin 26 g/l
Serum globulin 44 g/l
Alkaline phosphatase 125 u/l
Total bilirubin 66 μmol/l
  Direct 40
  Indirect 26
ALT 120 u/l
AST 130 u/l

Questions

1 Give four steps to manage hepatic encephalopathy for an elderly patient.
2 What is the most likely diagnosis in this patient?
3 What is the likely cause of hypokalaemia?
4 What five investigations will you ask for?
5 Name five common precipitating causes of hepatic encephelopathy.

Answers to case 19

1 (a) Protein restriction
(b) Cathartic/enemas to clear the bowels of its nitrogenous contents
(c) Oral neomycin to reduce bacterial flora of the gut
(d) Lactulose to produce osmotic diarrhoea

2 The most likely diagnosis in this patient is cirrhosis of the liver. Features of cirrhosis in this patient include jaundice, spider naevi, palmar erythema, pitting oedema, evidence of portal hypertension, (splenomegaly, ascites and dilated abdominal veins) with hypo-

albuminaemia and raised serum enzymes. Two pints of beer a day is unlikely to result in alcoholic cirrhosis. Crytogenic (idiopathic) cirrhosis is a likely possibility in this patient.

3 Secondary aldosteronism in cirrhosis is commonly responsible for low serum potassium levels. Hypokalaemia in this patient has been further potentiated by the use of loop diuretics such as frusemide.

4 (a) Australia antigen
(b) Liver scan
(c) Barium swallow
(d) Serum alphafetoprotein
(e) Liver biopsy (after checking prothrombin)

5 (a) Gastrointestinal bleed
(b) Fluid, electrolyte imbalance
(c) Sedatives and tranquillizers
(d) Concurrent infections
(e) Protein-rich diet

CASE 20

A man of 68 was admitted with a 4-week history of progressive jaundice, dark-coloured urine and light-coloured stools. He had an almost constant dull ache in his right hypochondrium with occasional radiation in his back. He had poor appetite and a feeling of gastric fulness. He had lost 1 stone in weight over the past 4 weeks. He had frequent bowel motions for the past 6 days but with no blood or mucus. His doctor had treated him at home with paracetamol, vitamins and laxative for this 'bad attack of hepatitis'.

On examination he was pale and deeply jaundiced and emaciated. There was no clubbing or lymphadenopathy. Blood pressure was 130/70. Pulse was 74/min regular. His liver was 6 cm enlarged, hard, non-tender with an irregular surface and no bruit, but no other mass could be felt in the abdomen. There was no ascites. Respiratory, cardiovascular and neurological examination proved normal. A day after his admission he started complaining of left painful calf which the house officer thought was probably deep venous thrombosis. Haemoglobin was reported as 10.8 g/dl and the routine urine examination was reported as showing excessive bilirubin but no urobilinogen or glucose.

Results of various other investigations were as follows:

ESR 48 mm/1st hour
MCV 92 fl
Sodium 140 mmol/l
Potassium 2.4 mmol/l
Chloride 97 mmol/l
Bicarbonate 24 mmol/l
Blood glucose 7.8 mmol/l
Blood urea 4.9 mmol/l
Chest X-ray normal

Questions

1 What is his most likely diagnosis?
2 What four investigations will help the diagnosis?
3 Give three endocrinal disturbances which may be associated with carcinoma of pancreas.

Answers to case 20

1 The most likely diagnosis in this patient with progressive jaundice is obstructive jaundice, probably caused by carcinoma of the head of pancreas. Contrary to the widely held opinion, pain is commonly associated with pancreatic carcinoma.

2 (a) Liver function tests
(b) Abdominal ultrasound
(c) Barium meal and follow-through ('inverted 3' sign)
(d) Abdominal CT scan

3 (a) Inappropriate ADH secretion
(b) Inappropriate ACTH secretion
(c) Carcinoid syndrome

CASE 21

A 59-year-old man living alone was admitted with a 1-month history of shortness of breath on exertion, lethargy and easy fatiguability. There was no history of cough, expectoration, chest pain or haemoptysis. He had no headaches or visual disturbances. He had lost his appetite recently with a weight loss of 6 pounds in the past 4 weeks. Bowel habits had remained unchanged. Two weeks ago he had a mild attack of shingles affecting his left forehead with no eye involvement. There was no history of any significant previous illnesses.

On examination he was pale. There were palpable scattered non-matted lymph nodes in both axillae and neck. JVP was not raised. Blood pressure was 160/90. Pulse rate was 80/min regular. Thyroid was not enlarged and there was no clubbing. There were no Dupuytren's contractures. Heart was in sinus rhythm with a soft murmur at the apex radiating all over the precordial area. His respiratory system was normal. Liver was 3 cm enlarged, firm, non-tender and smooth. Spleen was 4 cm enlarged with no ascites. There were no abnormalities in the neurological examination.

His routine blood tests were reported as follows:

Haemoglobin 9.9 g/dl
WBC 63 $\times$ 10^9/l
Lymphocytes 68%
MCV 99 fl
Platelet count normal
ESR 34 mm/h
Sodium 139 mmol/l
Potassium 3.9 mmol/l
Chloride 101 mmol/l
Bicarbonate 24 mmol/l
Blood glucose 5.4 mmol/l
Blood urea 4.3 mmol/l
Creatinine 127 μmol/l
Total protein 53 g/l
Albumin 29 g/l
Serum bilirubin 18 μmol/l
Chest X-ray – Heart size within normal limits; no active lung lesion seen

Questions

1 What is the main likely diagnosis?
2 What three further investigations will you ask for?
3 Give five indications of cytotoxic therapy in chronic lymphatic leukaemia.

Answers to case 21

1 The most likely diagnosis in this man with anaemia, hepatomegaly, lymphadenopathy, raised white cell count with lymphocytosis is chronic lymphatic leukaemia.

2 (a) Bone marrow aspiration and biopsy
(b) Reticulocyte count
(c) Coombs test (if reticulocyte count is high)

3 (a) Rapidly enlarging spleen or lymph node
(b) Progressive anaemia
(c) Thrombocytopenia with bleeding problems
(d) Recurrent infections.
(e) Worsening constitutional symptoms, e.g. unexplained fever, weight loss, etc

CASE 22

A 28-year-old schoolteacher was sent to the hospital by his family doctor with a 3-week history of cervical lymphadenopathy, weakness, fatigue, night sweats and generalized pruritis. He had a poor appetite and had lost 6 pounds in weight over the past 3 weeks. There was no history of cough, expectoration, chest pain, urinary or bowel symptoms. He had never been outside the United Kingdom and enjoyed good health until his present illness. He did not smoke or drink.

On examination he was pale, temperature was 37.5°C. Blood pressure was 135/80. Pulse was 84/min regular. JVP was not raised and he had no clubbing, cyanosis or oedema. Lymph nodes were enlarged in the left anterior cervical region and left axilla. Examination of cardiovascular and respiratory systems proved normal. There was no hepatosplenomegaly or ascites. Examination of central nervous system was unremarkable.

The following were the results of various initial investigations:

Haemoglobin 11.9 g/dl
MCV 89 fl
WBC 11.9 × 10^9/l
Sodium 136 mmol/l
Potassium 4.1 mmol/l
Chloride 100 mmol/l
Bicarbonate 26 mmol/l
Blood urea 6.9 mmol/l
Blood glucose 5.8 mmol/l
Urine analysis normal
Chest X-ray normal
ECG normal
Mantoux test negative

Questions

1 What is the most likely diagnosis?
2 Give four further investigations which will help your diagnosis and further management.
3 Name four chemotherapeutic agents useful for Hodgkin's disease.

Answers to case 22

1 The most likely diagnosis in this young patient with lymphadenopathy, fatigue, night sweats, generalized pruritis, weight loss, pyrexia and negative Mantoux test is Hodgkin's disease.

2 (a) Lymph node biopsy
(b) Bone marrow aspiration and biopsy
(c) Laparotomy with splenectomy, open liver biopsy and sampling of periaortic lymph nodes
(d) Lymphangiogram.

3 (a) Mustine
(b) Vincristine
(c) Prednisolone
(d) Procarbazine

CASE 23

J.F., a man of 59, was admitted with 5 week history of diarrhoea with little abdominal pain. He had four to six loose motions a day with occasional blood but no mucus. In spite of normal appetite he had recently lost 4 pounds in weight and felt generally tired since the onset of diarrhoea. There was no history of similar illness in the past. He had smoked 10 cigarettes a day for the last 40 years.

On examination he was mildly anaemic and apyrexial. JVP was not raised. Blood pressure was 150/100, pulse was 88/min irregular. Thyroid was not enlarged and clubbing was nil. Respiratory system was normal except for occasional scattered rhonchi. He was fibrillating with an apical rate of 90/min, with no heart murmurs. Abdomen was soft with no tenderness. Bowel sounds were present. No hepatosplenomegaly. PR some external piles were seen, the rectum was empty. Sigmoidoscopy up to 20 cm was normal.

Initial results were as follows:

Haemoglobin 10.6 g/dl
ESR 54 mm/1st hour
MCV 74 fl
WBC 6.9 × 10^9/l
Sodium 137 mmol/l
Potassium 3.2 mmol/l
Chloride 96 mmol/l
Bicarbonate 26 mmol/l
Urea 8.9 mmol/l
Creatinine 147 μmol/l
Blood sugar 5.2 mmol/l

Three specimens of stools were sent for culture and sensitivity, ova and cyst. There were no ova or cyst seen but on the basis of stool culture report he was started on oral erythromycin. His diarrhoea settled within a few days of his treatment.

Questions

1 What is the most likely cause of his diarrhoea?
2 What another investigation would you ask for this patient?
3 Name three other bacterial infections which may cause diarrhoea.
4 What is the cause of his anaemia?

Answers to case 23

1 The most likely cause for his diarrhoea is **Campylobacter** *infection, which is a not an uncommon cause of diarrhoea, affecting people of all ages. This infection responds very well to erythromycin therapy.*

2 A barium enema examination is important to look for other lesions such as carcinoma of colon and diverticular disease, etc.

3 (a) **Clostridium difficile**
(b) **Salmonella**
(c) **Shigella**

4 His low haemoglobin (10.6 g/dl) with low MCV indicates chronic blood loss. The presence of piles is a common cause of such anaemia in adults. Bloody diarrhoea may also be a feature of **Campylobacter** *infection and result in anaemia.*

CASE 24

Mrs A.N., a 52-year-old part-time medical secretary, had been taking bronchodilators and prednisolone 5 mg daily for her late-onset chronic asthma, for the past 8 years. Following a recent cold her asthma worsened and her doctor increased the prednisolone to 20 mg daily. She was also given a course of Amoxil for 1 week. Her condition improved with this treatment but after 2 weeks, while she was still taking 12.5 mg of prednisolone a day, she started feeling unwell with persistent cough with mucoid phlegm, night sweats and poor appetite.

On examination in the surgery she looked ill. Temperature was 37.8°C, pulse 90/min regular, JVP not raised. BP 130/90. No clubbing. She had two small lymph nodes palpable in the left supraclavicular fossa. Respiratory system – she had poor expansion of chest with left basal crepitations and scattered rhonchi. Liver was 3 cm enlarged, smooth and non-tender. There was no splenomegaly or ascites. Cardiovascular and neurological examination proved normal.

Her doctor arranged for a chest X-ray which was reported as 'Bilateral patchy shadowing compatible with bronchopneumonia. Heart size is within normal limits.'

She was given a trial of erythromycin for a week but with little benefit. She had lost half a stone in weight during this week and was admitted for urgent investigations.

Blood investigations on admission were as follows:

Haemoglobin 8.4 g/dl
WBC 11 × 10^9/l
Neutrophils 58%
Lymphocytes 20%
Monocytes 18%
Eosinophils 4%
ESR 110 mm/1st hour
MCV 79 fl
Platelets 120,000/mm^3
Urea 4.9 mmol/l
Sodium 134 mmol/l
Potassium 4.1 mmol/l
Chlorine 100 mmol/l
Bilirubin 17 μmol/l
Total protein 63 g/l
Albumin 27 g/l

Questions

1 What is the most likely diagnosis?
2 What four further investigations will help the diagnosis?

Answers to case 24

1 The most likely diagnosis in this 52-year-old secretary with cough, expectoration, malaise, pyrexia, loss of weight, hepatomegaly and lymphadenopathy, anaemia, monocytosis and very high ESR is miliary tuberculosis. The fact that she had been taking prednisolone over a long period of time makes the possibility of tuberculosis much stronger.

2 (a) *Mantoux test (this may be negative in miliary tuberculosis)*
(b) *Bone marrow aspiration and biopsy for culture*
(c) *Liver biopsy*
(d) *Lymph node biopsy*

CASE 25

A 69-year-old man was admitted after a sudden collapse in the street. There was no history of chest pain, palpitation, cough, expectoration, urinary or bowel symptoms. He had previously been fit and had no history of headaches, fits or faints. He had never 'bothered' his doctor in his life. He had been smoking 20 cigarettes a day for over 35 years but took alcohol only occasionally.

On examination he was conscious and mentally alert. Blood pressure was 90/70, pulse was 98/min regular with occasional ectopics; thyroid and lymph nodes were not enlarged; no anaemia, clubbing, cyanosis or jaundice. His apex beat was in the fifth intercostal space inside the midclavicular line. He had triple rhythm but no heart murmurs.

Examination of respiratory system, abdomen and nervous system was unremarkable.

The following were the results of various investigations:

Haemoglobin 13.4 g/dl
WBC 9.4 × 10^9/l
ESR 34 mm/1st hour
Sodium 136 mmol/l
Potassium 3.5 mmol/l
Chloride 100 mmol/l
Bicarbonate 25 mmol/l
Blood urea 9 mmol/l
Chest X-ray – Unfolding of aorta; heart size within normal limits

Questions

1 What is the most likely diagnosis?
2 What two investigations will help the diagnosis?
3 Give various atypical presentations of myocardial infarction in the elderly.

Answers to case 25

1 The most likely diagnosis in this elderly man with sudden collapse, low blood pressure, rapid pulse with extrasystole and triple rhythm is acute myocardial infarction. Myocardial infarction in the elderly may be completely silent and without any chest pain.

2 (a) ECG
(b) Cardiac enzymes

3 (a) Silent infarction
(b) Sudden confusional state
(c) Sudden dyspnoea
(d) Syncope
(e) Vomiting and sudden unexplained deterioration in general health
(f) Thromboembolism, e.g. stroke

CASE 26

A 70-year-old man was admitted with a 1-day history of worsening dyspnoea on exertion without any associated chest pain. He had had mild chronic obstructive airways disease for the past 10 years but had felt better for the past 2 months since stopping smoking. He had some white mucoid phlegm with cough but no haemoptysis. There was no history of loss of weight and appetite, urinary or bowel symptoms. He had increased his 'breathing tablets' from two to three but this had not helped the breathing.

On examination he was dyspnoeic. There was no cyanosis, clubbing or lymphadenopathy. Blood pressure 140/70. Pulse 88/min regular. JVP was not raised, no ankle oedema. Peripheral pulses were palpable. His trachea was shifted somewhat to the left. He had limited chest expansion, hyperresonance on percussion in the right upper zone with absent breath sounds. 'Coin sign' was positive. There were widespread rhonchi all over the chest. Apex beat was in the fifth intercostal space 3 cm outside the midclavicular line but his heart was in sinus rhythm. Abdomen and nervous system examination proved normal.

Results of various investigations were as follows:

Haemoglobin 13.4 g/dl
ESR 29 mm/1st hour
Urea 4.3 mmol/l
Blood sugar 7.6 mmol/l
Sodium 144 mmol/l
Potassium 3.5 mmol/l
Chloride 100 mmol/l
Bicarbonate 24 mmol/l
WBC 7.9×10^9/l
Polymorph 60%
Lymphocyte 38%
Eosinophils 2%
Total protein 60 g/l
Albumin 32 g/l
Bilirubin 16 μmol/l
ECG – No infarction; evidence of mild right ventricular hypertrophy seen

Questions

1 What is the diagnosis?
2 What two further investigations will you ask for?
3 Give four important causes of pneumothorax.

Answers to case 26

1 The most likely diagnosis in this elderly gentleman with previous history of chronic obstructive airways disease, worsening dyspnoea in the absence of any obvious exacerbation of chronic bronchitis with shifting of his trachea and apex beat, hyperresonant percussion note and positive 'coin test' is right pneumothorax.

2 (a) Chest X-ray
(b) Sputum for cytology, AFB, culture and sensitivity

3 (a) Spontaneous pneumothorax
(b) Carcinoma lung
(c) Pulmonary tuberculosis
(d) Trauma to the chest wall

CASE 27

J.C., a 68-year-old lady, was referred to the clinic with a 1-week history of diplopia. Three years ago she had a mild cerebrovascular accident with left-sided hemiparesis which recovered well. Two years ago she had started to suffer grand mal epileptic fits which were thought to be as a result of her previous stroke. The fits had been well controlled on phenytoin 300 mg a day. Two weeks ago she contracted shingles, affecting her left forehead. She denied any past history of headaches or vomiting. She lived alone and had good neighbours. She was frequently visited by her daughter who lived 10 miles away from her.

On examination she was mentally alert and could walk with the help of her stick. She had some scarring of her left forehead. Blood pressure was 160/110, pulse 74/min regular. There was no anaemia or clubbing. Thyroid was not enlarged and the lymph glands were not palpable. Cardiovascular, respiratory systems and abdomen were normal. Her left eye was pulled medially and she had paralytic strabismus of her sixth (abducent) cranial nerve, failed to move her left eye when asked to look towards her left, and complained of double vision. The rest of the eye movements were normal. Light and accommodation reflexes in both eyes were normal. Fundi were normal on both sides. Apart from mild residual weakness of the left side resulting from previous stroke there were no new neurological signs. CT brain scan was reported as showing no evidence of space-occupying lesion.

Questions

1 What is the diagnosis?
2 What are the other causes of diplopia?

Answers to case 27

1 The diagnosis is paralytic squint due to left sixth nerve palsy causing diplopia. In this patient this abducent palsy was probably a sequela of anterior horn cell involvement with herpes zoster.

2 (a) Abnormal neuromuscular function caused by: vascular lesion; neoplasm; infective, e.g. encephalitis; or degenerative disorder e.g. disseminated sclerosis
(b) Myasthenia gravis
(c) Ocular myopathy

CASE 28

A 43-year-old lady was referred to the outpatient clinic with a 4-month history of painless swelling of her thyroid gland. She had otherwise been very fit and healthy and denied any difficulties with her speech, swallowing or breathing. She had good appetite and had not lost any weight recently. There was no history of chest pain, palpitation, cough, expectoration or urinary or bowel disturbance.

On examination she looked fit. JVP was normal. There was no anaemia, clubbing, tremor or lymphadenopathy. Blood pressure was 140/70 and pulse was 74/min regular. She had a solitary thyroid nodule 2 × 2 cm firm and non-tender. Apex beat was in the fifth intercostal space inside the midclavicular line. She was in sinus rhythm and had no murmurs. Examination of central nervous system, respiratory system and abdomen proved normal.

Blood results were as follows:

Haemoglobin 13.4 g/dl
WBC 10 × 10^9/l
ESR 29 mm/1st hour
Sodium 140 mmol/l
Potassium 4.2 mmol/l
Chloride 96 mmol/l
Bicarbonate 22 mmol/l
Urea 6 mmol/l
Blood glucose 4.9 mmol/l
Total protein 72 g/l
Albumin 34 g/l
Bilirubin 12 μmol/l

Questions

1 What is the most likely diagnosis?
2 What three investigations will help in the management?
3 If her thyroid function is normal, how would you manage a solitary 'cold' nodule?

Answers to case 28

1 On the basis of history and clinical examination this lady is clinically euthyroid. She has a solitary thyroid nodule. It is important to confirm through further investigations that her thyroid function is normal. Further tests are also required to establish whether this nodule is benign or malignant.

2 (a) Serum thyroxine (T4), tri-iodothyronine (T_3) estimation
(b) Radioisotope scan
(c) Needle biopsy

3 Since up to 50 per cent of the solitary nodules subjected to surgery are found to be multinodular goitres and up to 2 per cent of these are due to thyroid carcinoma, surgical exploration and resection of such nodule is advisable.

CASE 29

A man of 62 was referred to the medical outpatient department with a history of swelling over his right elbow which he had noticed about 4 weeks ago. He denied any history of trauma. In the past he had always had good health and had been living alone since the death of his wife 3 years ago. He smoked 10 cigarettes a day and had had 1–2 pints of beer most evenings for many years.

On examination he was obese, his blood pressure was 180/100, pulse 78/min regular, JVP was normal. There was no clubbing, thyroid or lymph node enlargement. The swelling overlying his olecranon was about 2 cm, soft, non-tender and fluctuant. The temperature and the colour of the overlying skin was normal, movements of the elbow joint were normal and examination of the other joints was normal. Over his left ear he was noted to have two small tophi. His heart was in sinus rhythm with apex beat localized in the fifth intercostal space inside the midclavicular line. Trachea was central with normal chest expansion and air entry. There was no hepatosplenomegaly. Examination of central nervous system was unremarkable.

The following were the results of various investigations:

Haemoglobin 12.8 g/dl
Total protein 68 g/l
Albumin 38 g/l
Bilirubin 12 pmol/l
Sodium 139 mmol/l
Potassium 4.1 mmol/l
Chloride 99 mmol/l
Bicarbonate 24 mmol/l
Blood glucose 5.9 mmol/l
Blood urea 4.2 mmol/l
Chest X-ray normal

Questions

1 What is the most likely diagnosis, and why?
2 What are the other common causes of bursitis?
3 What three investigations would you ask for?
4 Name four commonly associated conditions with primary gout?
5 Name three drugs which are commonly used for the treatment of chronic gout?

Answers to case 29

1 The most likely diagnosis is gouty olecranon bursitis. The presence of gouty tophi over the left ear is highly suggestive of chronic gout.

2 (a) Traumatic
(b) Septic
(c) Rheumatoid arthritis

3 (a) Estimation of serum uric acid
(b) Aspiration of the swelling
(c) Rheumatoid factor

4 *(a)* ***Obesity***
(b) ***Diabetes mellitus***
(c) ***Hypertension***
(d) ***Ischaemic heart disease***

5 *(a)* ***Allopurinol***
(b) ***Probenecid***
(c) ***Sulphinpyrazone***

CASE 30

A 38-year-old married man was admitted with an 8-hour history of mid-epigastric pain, nausea and vomiting. The pain was localized, severe and almost constant in intensity, and was somewhat relieved on leaning forward. He had three vomitings consisting of undigested food and liquid but no blood. Before being sent to the hospital he had tried three doses of Milk of Magnesia but they did not help. He had enjoyed good health and had no previous significant illnesses. He smoked 25 cigarettes a day and drank 4–5 pints of beer every day.

On examination he was uncomfortable and in pain. Blood pressure was 110/70. Pulse was 98/min regular. JVP was not raised. There was no anaemia, cyanosis, jaundice, clubbing or oedema and all his peripheral pulses were palpable. He had marked epigastric tenderness with rigidity. Bowel sounds were audible. Liver and spleen were not palpable and there was no ascites. Examination of cardiovascular, respiratory and central nervous systems proved normal.

Results of various initial investigations were as follows:

Haemoglobin 12.4 g/dl
MCV 88 fl
WBC 9.8 × 10^9/l
Sodium 139 mmol/l
Potassium 3.4 mmol/l
Chloride 98 mmol/l
Bicarbonate 25 mmol/l
Urea 6 mmol/l
Random blood glucose 6.1 mmol/l
Serum amylase 750 Somogyi units
Chest X-ray normal
X-ray abdomen – No air under the diaphragm; no fluid levels seen
ECG – Sinus tachycardia
Urine analysis – Trace protein; no sugar

Questions

1 What is the differential diagnosis in this patient?
2 What five further investigations will you ask for?

Answers to case 30

1 The differential diagnosis in this patient with prolonged epigastric pain, nausea and vomiting, history of moderately heavy smoking and alcohol intake is peptic ulcer disease, acute pancreatitis or cholecystitis. Radiation of the pain to the back in pancreatitis, and to the right hypochondrium or to the right shoulder in cholecystitis, certainly helps in the diagnosis. Yet at times in both these conditions the pain may remain localized to the epigastrium. A significantly raised serum amylase level, as is the case in this patient, is suggestive of the diagnosis of acute pancreatitis.

2 (a) Urinary amylase estimation
(b) Serum calcium and phosphorus
(c) Liver function test
(d) Barium meal at a later stage
(e) Serum cholesterol and triglycerides

CASE 31

A 68-year-old gentleman was admitted with 2 week history of progressive confusion, increasing cough and mucopurulent expectoration. There was no history of chest pain, palpitation or haemoptysis. His appetite remained unchanged and he had not lost any weight. There were no urinary or bowel symptoms. He had been 'chesty' for over 20 years and smoked 30 cigarettes a day for as long as he could remember.

On examination he was dyspnoeic and centrally cyanosed. JVP was raised by 3 cm and he had moderate pitting oedema over both his legs. Blood pressure 140/90. Pulse was 98/min regular. There was no clubbing, jaundice or lymphadenopathy. Hearts sounds were normal except for a loud and accentuated P2. There were no heart murmurs. His chest was barrel-shaped with limited expansion. Vocal fremitus and percussion notes were normal with vesicular breathing but he had scattered rhonchi and bilateral basal crepitations. Liver was 3 cm enlarged, smooth and tender. There was no ascites or splenomegaly. He was moderately confused and disorientated. Fundi and cranial nerves were normal and there were no localizing neurological signs.

The following were the results of various initial investigations:

Haemoglobin 17 g/dl
MCV 82 fl
WBC 14.8 × 10^9/l
Polymorphs 78%
Lymphocytes 21%
Eosinophils 1%
Sodium 138 mmol/l
Potassium 3.9 mmol/l
Chloride 98 mmol/l
Bicarbonate 28 mmol/l
Blood urea 8.3 mmol/l
Random blood glucose 4.9 mmol/l
Chest X-ray – Emphysematous lung fields with patchy shadowing right base

Questions

1 What is the most likely diagnosis?
2 What three further investigations will you ask for?
3 Give six important steps in the management of this patient.

Answers to case 31

1 The most likely diagnosis in this gentleman with chronic bronchitis (being chesty and a heavy smoker), raised JVP, hepatomegaly, pitting ankle oedema, cyanosis, dyspnoea, confusion, high white cell count with polymorph leucocytosis is acute on chronic bronchitis, chronic cor pulmonale and probable respiratory failure.

2 (a) Arterial blood gases
(b) Sputum for culture and sensitivity
(c) ECG

3 (a) Oxygen inhalation (low dose)
(b) Antibiotics
(c) Digoxin
(d) Diuretics
(e) Chest physiotherapy
(f) Consider assisted ventilation if blood gases confirm respiratory failure.

CASE 32

A man of 69 was admitted via the accident and emergency department with sudden onset of numbness and weakness of his left face, arm and leg. He also lost his speech. There was no history of loss of consciousness, convulsions or tongue-biting. He had a similar episode of weakness 3 months ago which lasted for only 5 minutes. There was no history of chest pain or palpitation.

On examination he was aphasic, blood pressure was 150/80, pulse 74/min regular. Thyroid was not enlarged and there was no clubbing or lymphadenopathy. Apex beat was in the fourth intercostal space. He was in sinus rhythm with no heart murmurs. There was a distinctly audible carotid bruit on the right side of his neck. Examination of respiratory system and abdomen proved normal. Cranial nerves, including fundi, were intact but he had diminished power and tone with absent tendon reflexes on his left side. The left plantar was upgoing. After 1 hour his numbness and weakness and speech difficulty improved dramatically.

Initial investigations were as follows:

Haemoglobin 13.4 g/dl
WBC 10×10^9/l
ECG – mild ischaemic changes in left chest leads
Chest X-ray – No lung lesion; heart size normal
BM Stix 6 mmol

Questions

1 What is the most likely diagnosis?
2 How can you confirm the diagnosis?
3 What three drugs are commonly used for transient ischaemic attack?
4 What are the risks of not treating such patients?

Answers to case 32

1 The most likely diagnosis in this elderly patient with sudden onset of numbness and weakness affecting his left side with right carotid bruit with dramatic improvement within 1 hour (with no therapy) is transient ischaemic attack, probably caused by right carotid artery stenosis.

2 Carotid angiography to demonstrate the degree of occlusion is the only confirmatory investigation.

3 (a) Dipyridamole (Persantin)
(b) Aspirin (300–600 mg daily)
(c) Anticoagulant such as warfarin

4 Patients with frequent transient ischaemic attacks are at risk of suffering complete strokes; therefore every effort must be made to control further transient ischaemic attacks.

CASE 33

J.R., a man of 74, a known diabetic controlled on chlorpropramide for over 6 years, was admitted with 8 hours history of confusion, sweating, aggressive behaviour, dizziness and left-sided weakness. He was well until the previous day and took his diabetic tablet in the morning on the day of admission but had missed his breakfast.

On examination he was disorientated. Blood pressure was 170/110, pulse 98/min regular. He was sweating profusely and was rather drowsy. Cardiovascular, respiratory and abdominal examination was normal. Cranial nerves were intact but he had weakness of his left upper and lower limbs. All tendon reflexes were brisk with bilateral plantar extensor responses.

Initial results were as follows:

Haemoglobin 12.8 g/dl
Sodium 137 mmol/l
Urea 7 mmol/l
Potassium 4.3 mmol/l
Chloride 99 mmol/l
Bicarbonate 24 mmol/l
Urine – No glucose or ketones
BM Stix 3 mmol

Questions

1 What is the most likely diagnosis?
2 Name three drugs that may be used for correction of hypoglycaemic state.

Answers to case 33

1 The most likely diagnosis in this elderly diabetic on long-acting oral hypoglycaemic agent admitted after missing his breakfast with sweating, dizziness, confusion, aggressive behaviour and left-sided weakness is hypoglycaemia. This is further confirmed by his low BM Stix (3 mmol) and absence of glycosuria.

2 (a) Glucose (preferably given intravenously).
(b) Glucagon (to be used only if the hypoglycaemia has been caused by insulin injection)
(c) Adrenaline

CASE 34

A man of 43 had flu-like illness which was treated by his GP with analgesics and a course of antibiotics. He felt better for the first 3 days but later started getting excessively tired, lost his appetite, and became generally unwell. He had difficulty in walking and took to his bed. His wife reported that he could not swallow his food. He was therefore admitted to the medical unit for further investigation and treatment.

On examination he was mentally alert. JVP was not raised. There was no clubbing or lymphadenopathy. Blood pressure was 130/70 pulse was 78/min regular. Cardiovascular system, respiratory system and abdomen were normal. He had weakness of all four limbs with reduced tone and absent tendon reflexes. Plantars were unequivocal. There was some loss of touch and pain sensation in both lower limbs below the knees. All cranial nerves except ninth and tenth were normal.

Blood investigations were as follows:

Haemoglobin 11.7 g/dl
MCV 87 fl
WBC 4×10^9/l
ESR 46 mm/1st hour
Sodium 142 mmol/l
Potassium 4.3 mmol/l
Chloride 99 mmol/l
Bicarbonate 28 mmol/l
Urea 4.9 mmol/l
Total bilirubin 16 μmol/l
Total protein 70 g/l

Questions

1 What is the most likely diagnosis?
2 What four investigations will you ask for?
3 What is the role of steroids in the treatment?

Answers to case 34

1 The most likely diagnosis in this man with acute onset of progressive weakness of all four limbs, and swallowing difficulty preceded by a flu-like illness, is acute polyneuropathy (Guillain–Barré syndrome).

2 (a) Lumbar puncture (very high protein with no cells in cerebrospinal fluid)
(b) Nerve conduction studies
(c) Lung function test, e.g. spirometry
(d) Viral studies.

3 Steroids have been used for many years but recent studies have not only failed to show any benefit, but have raised fears about delayed recovery and long-term complications in patients treated with steroids.

CASE 35

P.C., a 69-year-old man, was admitted with 2 month history of upper abdominal pain, anorexia and weight loss of 1 stone. For the past 2 weeks he had started vomiting but there was no haematemesis. He had been taking antacid and cimetidine with some relief for the first few days only. There was no history of cough, expectoration, bowel or urinary disturbance.

He lived alone in a flat and had meals-on-wheels, which he never fancied much. He had stopped going to the nearby day centre for the past 5 weeks since he felt too weak.

On examination he was pale, frail and emaciated. JVP was not raised. He had a palpable left supraclavicular lymph node but no thyroid enlargement, clubbing or oedema. There were no spider naevi or palmar erythema. His liver was 3 cm enlarged, hard, nodular and non-tender. Spleen was not palpable. There was no ascites, other masses or tenderness. Rectal examination was normal. Respiratory and cardiovascular systems, and neurological examination, proved normal. A day after his admission he developed deep venous thrombosis of his left calf.

Blood results were as follows:

Haemoglobin 8.2 g/dl
Total protein 54 g/l
Albumin 26 g/l
Bilirubin 28 μmol/l
AST 38 u/l
Alkaline phosphatase 249 u/l
WBC 4.9 × 10^9/l
ESR 74 mm/1st hour
Stools – Occult blood positive on two occasions

Questions

1 What is the most likely diagnosis?
2 What three further investigations will you arrange for?
3 Why did the patient improve initially with cimetidine?

Answers to case 35

1 The most likely diagnosis in this elderly gentleman with upper abdominal pain, anorexia, weight loss, vomiting, left supraclavicular lymphadenopathy, hard nodular liver enlargement with some initial response to cimetidine therapy is carcinoma of stomach with secondaries in the liver.

2 (a) Barium meal
(b) Upper gastrointestinal endoscopy
(c) Lymph node/liver biopsy

3 An H_2 antagonist such as cimetidine has been known to temporarily improve the symptoms in patients with gastric carcinoma and therefore indiscriminate use of cimetidine without establishing proper diagnosis with barium meal/endoscopy is not encouraged, and can in fact be very misleading.

CASE 36

A 62-year-old lady was admitted with a 3-day history of burning sensation over her left forehead and eye. Her doctor did not find any visible lesion and she was sent in as an atypical case of facial pain. A day after her admission she had papular rash all over her left forehead limited to the midline. She was apyrexial. Blood pressure was 170/90 and pulse was 80/min regular. There was no thyroid enlargement but she had palpable lymph nodes in her neck and both axillae and left preauricular region. She had no anaemia or clubbing. Spleen was 4 cm enlarged but the liver was not palpable, nor was there any evidence of ascites. Cardiovascular, respiratory and neurological examination proved normal.

Over the next few days the papular rashes developed into vesicles which became dry and crusty. Since her left eye pain continued she was seen by an ophthalmologist who noticed a small superficial left corneal ulcer with keratitis. She was given two types of eye drops for her eye problem.

Questions

1 What is the diagnosis?
2 What three investigations will you ask for?
3 What were the likely eye drops supplied by the Ophthalmologist?
4 Name four agents which may prevent or help in treating post herpetic neuralgia.

Answers to case 36

1 The diagnosis in this elderly lady with left facial pain, rashes limited to the left half of the forehead progressing through vesicles and crust and also involving her left eye, is herpes zoster (shingles) with ophthalmic involvement. Her left preauricular lymphadenopathy is probably a result of shingles, but the axillary and cervical lymphadenopathy with splenomegaly is suggestive of an underlying lymphoma, carcinomatosis or leukaemia.

2 (a) Haemoglobin full blood count and ESR
(b) Chest X-ray
(c) Lymph node biopsy

3 (a) Local steroids
(b) Mydriatrics

4 (a) Local iodoxuridine (Herpid) cream
(b) Local steroid cream
(c) Analgesic
(d) Carbamazepine

CASE 37

Mrs A.P., a 70-year-old lady, living alone, was referred to the medical outpatient clinic by her doctor. Her family doctor had recently seen her at home at the request of the home help. The home help had reported that the patient had been becoming progressively confused and less co-operative for the last 8 months. The home help had recently increased her visits to three times a week and had noticed that Mrs A.P. had been losing all interest in her surroundings; she would sit for hours in her chair and do nothing. She was becoming increasingly forgetful and had in fact forgotten to switch the gas off on at least on three occasions during the past 4 weeks.

On examination she was found to be pleasantly confused. Her blood pressure was 170/105. Pulse was 78/min regular. There was no anaemia, cyanosis, jaundice, oedema, thyroid or lymph node enlargement. Examination of cardiovascular and respiratory systems and abdomen proved normal. She could not remember the day, date or the month of the year. She could, however, remember her name, her own address and date of birth. She seemed to talk to herself from time to time while sitting in the outpatients. There were no focal neurological signs.

Questions

1 What is the likely diagnosis?
2 What is the incidence of dementia in old age?
3 What are the treatable causes of dementia?

Answers to case 37

1 The most likely diagnosis in this elderly lady with history of progressive self-neglect, confusion and forgetfulness is senile dementia, probably of Alzheimer type. Slow onset and progressive course of the disease are characteristic.

2 The incidence of dementia increases with ageing. It is estimated that about 5 per cent of the population over the age of 65 has dementia, but over the age of 80 the incidence is much higher and is about 20 per cent.

3 (a) Traumatic, e.g. subdural haematoma
(b) Vitamin deficiencies, e.g. B_1, B_{12} and folic acid deficiencies
(c) Metabolic causes, e.g. hypothyroidism, hypercalcaemia, Cushing's syndrome, chronic renal failure, hepatic encephalopathy
(d) Infections, e.g. neurosyphilis
(e) Neoplasms–brain tumour
(f) Others such as normal-pressure hydrocephalus

CASE 38

H.P., a 65-year-old man, was admitted with a 6 week history of purpuric, non-itchy rashes on his legs, thighs (extensor aspects) and buttocks. There was no history of preceding sore throat. For 3 days before admission he had bloody diarrhoea with central colicky abdominal pain but no vomiting or haematemesis. Sigmoidoscopy, rectal biopsy and barium enema was found to be normal. The bloody diarrhoea lasted 6 days in all. Urine examination revealed microscopic haematuria with granular red blood cell casts and mild proteinuria. A fortnight after admission he complained of painful mild swelling of both knees and left ankle. This was treated with paracetamol and subsided within a week.

Various blood results were as follows:

Haemoglobin 13.8 g/dl
WBC 9 × 10^9/l
Platelet count 260 × 10^9/l
Albumin 38 g/l
Urate 353 μmol/l
Alkaline phosphatase 50 u/l
Total bilirubin 9 μmol/l
Aspartate aminotransferase 301 u/l
Calcium 2.30 mmol/l
Phosphorus 0.87 mmol/l
Total protein 70 g/l

Questions

1 What is the most likely diagnosis?
2 What three further investigations will help the diagnosis?
3 What is the cause of haematuria in Henoch-Schönlein purpura?
4 What is the treatment of Henoch-Schönlein purpura?
5 What are two important complications of Henoch-Schönlein purpura?

Answers to case 38

1 The most likely diagnosis in this patient with purpuric spots, bloody diarrhoea, haematuria, and anthralgia with normal platelet count is Henoch–Schonlein purpura. Though the condition is seen most commonly in young children (median age 4 years) rarely the patient may by much older.

2 (a) Antistreptolysin O titre
(b) Serum complements assay
(c) Renal biopsy

3 Haematuria in these patients may be a consequence of bleeding from the mucosal surface of the ureters, bladder and urethra. More commonly the haematuria results from true glomerulonephritis.

4 There is no specific therapy available as yet. Steroids and immunosuppressive agents have been used. There is no definite evidence, however, that they have any beneficial effect.

5 (a) Hypertension
(b) Renal failure

CASE 39

A 70-year-old man was admitted with a 2-day history of continuous left lower abdominal pain. The pain was localized and there was no associated nausea or vomiting. He had had a tendency towards constipation for the past 6 months but had two bouts of diarrhoea which settled without any specific therapy. On two occasions he had passed fresh blood with the stools, about 4 weeks ago. He also complained of flatulence and heartburn for the past 3 months. There was no history of loss of appetite and his weight had remained steady for the past 20 years. There were no urinary symptoms.

On examination he was pyrexial with a temperature of 38°C, blood pressure was 140/90, pulse 88/min, thyroid and lymph nodes not enlarged. No clubbing, anaemia, jaundice or oedema. He had ill-defined tender left iliac fossa mass with no guarding. Rectal examination proved normal. Sigmoidoscopy was not performed because of his increasing pain and discomfort. There were no piles. Respiratory, cardiovascular and central nervous systems were normal.

Initial investigation results were as follows:

Haemoglobin 12.9 g/dl
Protein 67 g/l
Albumin 32 g/l
Urea 8 mmol/l
WBC 14 × 10^9/l
Sodium 142 mmol/l
Potassium 4.3 mmol/l
Chloride 100 mmol/l
Bicarbonate 24 mmol/l

Questions

1 What is the most likely diagnosis?
2 Name three complications of diverticular disease.
3 How would you manage this problem?

Answers to case 39

1 The most likely diagnosis in this elderly man with change of bowel habit, rectal bleeding, flatulence, heartburn and left lower abdominal pain with an ill defined tender mass and leucocytosis is acute diverticulitis. Diverticular disease of the colon is common in the elderly and if associated with complication may present as 'acute abdomen'.

2 (a) Acute diverticulitis with abscess
(b) Perforation and peritonitis
(c) Intestinal obstruction

3 His acute diverticulitis should be treated with rest, parenteral fluids, antibiotics and adequate pain control. After recovery a coexistent neoplasm should be excluded by sigmoidoscopy, barium enema and colonoscopy, if required.

CASE 40

A 43-year-old man had recently returned from a 2-week holiday in Spain and was admitted with 5 day history of flu-like symptoms, malaise, headaches, chest pain and unproductive cough. His doctor had started him on tetracycline but this had to be stopped after 2 days because he was getting worse.

For the past 3 days he had taken ampicillin, without any benefit. In the past he had always been fit and healthy. There were no other significant systemic symptoms.

He lived with his wife near Nottingham and had a small business which they had jointly looked after for over 10 years.

On examination he was confused, disorientated and dehydrated. Blood pressure was 150/85 pulse was 76/min, temperature 38°C. Thyroid and lymph nodes were not enlarged; there was no clubbing or oedema. Trachea was central, breath sounds were impaired at both bases with widespread crepitations but no pleural rub or bronchial breathing. Abdomen, cardiovascular and respiratory systems were normal.

The following results were available within 3 hours of his admission:

Haemoglobin 13.9 g/dl
ESR 69 mm/1st hour
Urea 4.8 mmol/l
Sodium 139 mmol/l
Potassium 4.1 mmol/l
Chloride 98 mmol/l
Bicarbonate 23 mmol/l
WBC 8.9 × 10^9/l
Polymorphs 92%
Lymph 7%
Eosinophils 1%
Blood sugar 5.5 mmol/l

Questions

1 What is the most likely diagnosis?
2 What four investigations will you ask for?
3 Name two antibiotics helpful in the treatment of Legionnaire's disease.

Answers to case 40

1 The most likely diagnosis in this 43-year-old patient with clinical features of pneumonia with no response to tetracycline and ampicillin is some form of atypical pneumonia, e.g. Legionnaire's disease. Mycoplasma pneumonia is a possibility but mycoplasma pneumonia more commonly affects younger adults and usually responds to tetracycline therapy.

2 (a) Chest X-ray
(b) Sputum for culture and sensitivity
(c) Blood culture
(d) Serology – to look for rising titre of specific antibodies

3 (a) Erythromycin
(b) Rifampicin

CASE 41

A 60-year-old man was admitted with history of progressive cough mucoid phlegm and haemoptysis for the past 3 weeks. He had smoked 20 cigarettes a day for over 40 years and had a smoker's cough in the morning for over 13 years.

He had been unsuccessfully treated with a course of broad-spectrum antibiotic by his own doctor before being sent to the hospital. He had a good appetite and had not lost any weight recently. There was no history of chest pain, palpitation, urinary or bowel probelms.

On examination he looked fit. JVP was not raised. There was no anaemia, cyanosis, lymph node or thyroid enlargement. He had early clubbing of his fingers, more marked on the left side. Trachea was central. He had an area of bronchial breathing with few crepitations at his right base. Examination of cardiovascular system, abdomen and nervous system proved unremarkable. A day after his admission he had a grand mal epileptic fit.

Blood investigations were as follows:

Haemoglobin 11.4 g/dl
WBC 9.7 × 9^{10}/l
ESR 39 mm/1st hour
Urea 4.9 mmol/l
Sodium 139 mmol/l
Potassium 4.1 mmol/l
Chloride 101 mmol/l
Blood sugar 6 mmol/l

Questions

1 What is the likely diagnosis?
2 Give four investigations to help the diagnosis.
3 Give four 'endocrinopathies' which may be associated with carcinoma of lung.
4 Give two major contraindications for surgical resection in a patient with carcinoma of bronchus.

Answers to case 41

1 The most likely diagnosis in this man, who has been a moderately heavy smoker with cough, haemoptysis, clubbing, bronchial breathing and epileptic fit, is carcinoma of bronchus with brain metastasis.

2 (a) Chest X-ray
(b) Sputum cytology, culture sensitivity and AFB
(c) Bronchoscopy
(d) CT brain scan

3 (a) Hypercalcaemia
(b) Inappropriate ADH secretion
(c) Inappropriate ACTH secretion
(d) Carcinoid syndrome

4 (a) Inadequate ventilatory function (FEV_1 below 60 per cent of predicted value)
(b) Evidence of metastasis, e.g. in pleura, liver, brain, bone, etc.

CASE 42

A 72-year-old man was admitted with a 1-week history of cough, purulent phlegm, pleuritic chest pain, confusion and urinary incontinence. His bowels were normal and he had not lost any weight recently. He lived with his wife and had never been confused in the past. Four weeks ago he was started on carbamazepine for his trigeminal neuralgia.

On examination he was confused and disorientated and thought that he was still at home. Blood pressure was 140/80 mm lying and 130/75 mm on standing. Pulse 80/min regular; temperature 37°C. JVP was not raised and he had no clubbing oedema or dehydration. Cardiovascular and abdominal examination proved normal. He had signs of right basal consolidation with bronchial breathing and coarse crepitations but no pleural rub. Central nervous system (apart from his confusion) was normal.

Initial results were as follows:

Haemoglobin 12 g/dl
WBC 14 × 10^9/l
Polymorphs 89%
Lymphocytes 9%
Eosinophils 2%
Sodium 119 mmol/l
Potassium 4.1 mmol/l
Chloride 99 mmol/l
Bicarbonate 24 mmol/l
Urea 8 mmol/l
ESR 59 mm/1st hour
Blood sugar 6.9 mmol/l
Urine analysis normal

Questions

1 What is his most likely diagnosis?
2 What three investigations will you ask for in this patient?
3 Name four other drugs which may cause inappropriate ADH secretion.
4 Give four respiratory conditions which may be associated with inappropriate ADH secretion.

Answers to case 42

1 The most likely diagnosis in this elderly man with cough, expectoration, confusion, right basal consolidation and hyponatraemia in the absence of clinical dehydration is pneumonia with syndrome of inappropriate antidiuretic hormone secretion. Further, his hyponatraemia may be a result of carbamazepine therapy. He has two obvious causes of acute confusional state, i.e. pneumonia and hyponatraemia.

2 (a) Chest X-ray
(b) Plasma and urinary osmolality
(c) Bronchoscopy

3 (a) Chlorpropamide
(b) Thiazide diuretics
(c) Phenothiazines
(d) Tricyclic antidepressants

4 (a) Pneumonia
(b) Carcinoma of lung (oat-cell type, specially)
(c) Pulmonary tuberculosis
(d) Positive pressure ventilation

CASE 43

A 62-year-old retired bank clerk was admitted with a 4-month history of progressive shortness of breath on exertion. There was no history of wheezing or diurnal variation. For the past month she had started having an unproductive cough and 2 weeks ago she had arthralgia of her ankle and knee joints which settled with paracetamol tablets within 3 days. There was no history of chest pain, loss of weight or appetite.

She lived alone and had no pets at home. She had had ulcerative colitis for the past 18 years but for the past 3 years her colitis had been quiet and she was not taking any drugs.

On examination she was dyspnoeic and centrally cyanosed. She had marked clubbing of her fingers but had no enlargement of lymph nodes or thyroid. Blood pressure 160/90, pulse 88/min regular. She had pitting oedema of both her ankles and her JVP was raised by 3 cm. Skin was normal with no subcutaneous nodules or ulceration. Trachea was central but her chest expansion was limited and she had bilateral fine inspiratory crepitations over her lung bases. She was in sinus rhythm but had left parasternal heave and a loud pulmonary component of her second heart sound. Her liver was 3 cm enlarged, soft and tender with no associated splenomegaly or ascites. Examination of the nervous system proved normal.

The following investigation results were available:

Haemoglobin 13.9 g/dl
ESR 42 mm/1st hour
Sodium 139 mmol/l
Potassium 3.4 mmol/l
Chloride 96 mmol/l
Bicarbonate 27 mmol/l
WBC 8 × 10^9/l
Peak flow 200
Blood glucose 6.7 mmol/l
Total protein 62 g/l
Albumin 33 g/l
Bilirubin 16 μmol/l

Questions

1 What is the most likely diagnosis?
2 What five investigations will help the diagnosis?
3 Name five diseases known to be associated with cryptogenic fibrosing alveolitis.

Answers to case 43

1 The most likely diagnosis in this lady with progressive dyspnoea, no wheezing or diurnal variation, unproductive cough, central cyanois, clubbing and bilateral fine basal crepitations is idiopathic (cryptogenic) fibrosing alveolitis. Findings of left parasternal heave with loud P_2, raised JVP, ankle oedema and hepatomegaly suggest chronic cor pulmonale.

2 (a) Chest X-ray
(b) Lung function test (restrictive lung disorder and reduced CO diffusing capacity)
(c) Antinuclear antibodies
(d) Blood gases (low Po_2 and Pco_2)
(e) Lung biopsy

3 (a) ***Systemic lupus erythematosus***
(b) ***Rheumatoid arthritis***
(c) ***Dermato/polymyositis***
(d) ***Ulcerative colitis***
(e) ***Systemic sclerosis***

CASE 44

A 62-year-old lady was referred to the medical outpatient clinic with 8 month history of pruritus. She had had loose motions for the past 4 weeks and felt generally tired. There was no history of loss of weight or appetite. She had been applying calamine lotion over her skin but with little relief, though her diarrhoea was a little better with kaolin and morph given by her doctor 2 days ago.

On examination she was mildly icteric and had clubbing of her fingers. There was no lymphadenopathy or glandular enlargement. Blood pressure was 170/160. Pulse rate was 80/min. Her skin was a little dry and pigmented and she had scratch marks all over her body with bilateral xanthelasma. Respiratory and cardiovascular system were normal. Abdomen – liver was 6 cm enlarged, firm and smooth. The spleen was 3 cm enlarged and she had some shifting dullness but no definite fluid thrill could be elicited. Neurological examination proved normal.

Her initial blood results were as follows:

Haemoglobin 11 g/dl
WBC 9 × 10^9/l
Total bilirubin 26 μmol/l
  Direct 8 μmol/l
  Indirect 18 μmol/l
Protein 68 g/l
Albumin 38 g/l
MCV 86 fl
ESR 55 mm/h
AST 48 u/l
AP 130 u/l
GGT 70 u/l

Questions

1 What is the most likely diagnosis?
2 What four investigations will help the diagnosis?
3 How would you treat the pruritus?
4 What is secondary biliary cirrhosis?
5 What is Zieve's syndrome?
6 What is the prognosis of primary biliary cirrhosis?

Answers to case 44

1 The most likely diagnosis in this elderly lady with prolonged pruritis, jaundice with hepatosplenomegaly and xanthelasma is primary biliary cirrhosis.

2 (a) Serum cholesterol level (high)
(b) Antimitochondrial antibodies
(c) Serum IgM level (raised)
(d) Liver biopsy (after correction of prothrombin time)

3 If the obstruction is incomplete, cholestyramine 10–12 g daily in divided doses is helpful in controlling pruritus. Cholestyramine, by binding bile acids in the gut, increases their excretion. In complete biliary obstruction hormonal treatment with norethandrolone may be tried.

4 Secondary biliary cirrhosis is characterized by obstruction of the large extrahepatic bile ducts which may be caused by impaction of gallstone or stricture formation.

5 ***Zieve's syndrome is characterized by alcoholic hepatitis, jaundice, haemolytic anaemia and hypercholesterolaemia. The condition is seen after a bout of alcoholic drinking and usually settles if the person stops drinking.***

6 ***Patients usually die between 4 and 5 years after their initial symptoms.***

CASE 45

A 72-year-old lady was admitted with a 3-month history of tiredness, shortness of breath on exertion, swelling of both legs and occasional short-lived palpitation. She denied having any chest pain. Her appetite had been good and she had not lost any weight. Bowels were normal and there were no urinary symptoms. Her daughter who lived nearby visited her almost every day and confirmed that her mother was sometimes listless and confused, and was not coping well at home.

On examination she looked tired and apathetic and was mildly confused. JVP was raised by 2 cm and she had bilateral pitting ankle oedema. Blood pressure was 160/80 sitting 155/75 standing, pulse 130/min irregular. Thyroid and lymph nodes were not enlarged. She had some fine tremor in both hands but there was no lid lag or exophthalmos. She had bilateral medium crepitations in her chest. Apex beat was in the fifth intercostal space inside the midclavicular line, apex rate was 140 irregular and she had a widespread soft systolic murmur. Abdomen was normal and there were no localizing neurological signs. She could walk without any help.

The following were the results of various investigations:

Haemoglobin 12.4 g/dl
ESR 29 mm/1st hour
Sodium 136 mmol/l
Potassium 3.4 mmol/l
Chloride 96 mmol/l
Bicarbonate 27 mmol/l
WBC 6.9 × 10^9/l
Blood urea 10 mmol/l
Blood glucose 6.7 mmol/l
Serum T_4 100 μg/l (normal 40–110 μg/l)
Serum T_3 3.2 μg/l (normal 0.7–2 μg/l)
ECG – Atrial fibrillation with some ischaemic changes; no infarction

Questions

1 What is the most likely diagnosis?
2 Give five causes of falsely high T_3 results.
3 Give five causes of falsely high T_4 results.

Answers to case 45

1 The most likely diagnosis in this elderly lady with tiredness, dyspnoea, palpitation, occasional confusion, fine tremor, raised JVP, oedema, rapid atrial fibrillation and raised serum T_3 but normal thyroxine (T_4) is T_3 toxicosis. Atypical presentation of thyrotoxicosis is common in the elderly and features such as diarrhoea, anxiety, weight loss, intolerance to hot weather, increased appetite and eye signs may be completely missing, thus making diagnosis difficult.

2 (a) Pregnancy
(b) Oestrogen therapy
(c) Phenothiazine therapy
(d) Clofibrate therapy
(e) Viral hepatitis

3 (a) Nephrotic syndrome
(b) Malnutrition
(c) Androgen therapy
(d) Steroid therapy
(e) After surgery or prolonged ill-health

CASE 46

J.C., a 70-year-old known bronchitic, was admitted with increasing cough and dyspnoea on exertion. His appetite was poor but he was not sure whether he had lost any weight recently. There was no history of chest pain, palpitation or paroxysmal nocturnal dyspnoea.

He lived in a warden-controlled flat and received daily meals-on-wheels and home help twice a week. He had smoked 20 cigarettes a day for over 35 years but for the past 6 months he had successfully reduced his smoking to only five cigarettes a day. He had a partial gastrectomy at the age of 57.

On examination he was dyspnoeic, JVP was normal, temperature 38°C, blood pressure was 170/100. Pulse 78/min regular. Thyroid nil, clubbing nil. Lymph nodes nil. His chest expansion was poor, trachea was central, air entry was fair but he had widespread rhonchi with bilateral coarse crepitations. Heart was in sinus rhythm with no murmur. Examination of the abdomen and central nervous system proved normal. A day after his admission he had haemoptysis.

Initial investigations were:

Haemoglobin 11 g/dl
WBC 9.7×10^9/l
MCV 89 fl
Creatinine 90 μmol/l
ESR 108 mm/1st hour
Urea 11.3 mmol/l
Sodium 139 mmol/l
Potassium 4.3 mmol/l
Chest X-ray – Bilateral basal patchy shadowing – consistent with bronchopneumonia and healed calcified nodes in right hilum and apex.

Questions

1 What is the diagnosis?
2 What three further investigations will you ask for?
3 What is the most serious side-effect of ethambutol in the elderly?

Answers to case 46

1 ***Acute exacerbation of chronic bronchitis is quite common but haemoptysis and a very high ESR should make one suspicious of pulmonary tuberculosis, which at present is largely a disease of the elderly and the immigrant community in the United Kingdom.***

2 ***(a) Sputum for AFB and malignant cells***
(b) Tuberculin test
(c) Tomography of right lung apex

3 ***Visual disturbance because of retrobulbar neuritis is the most serious side-effect in older patients with impaired renal function. Low doses should therefore be used in the elderly, and the patient should be advised and supervised at regular intervals. If ethambutol is stopped at an early stage the visual defect is reversible.***

CASE 47

A 69-year-old lady was admitted with 3-month history of bone pains, anorexia, constipation, occasional vomiting, easy fatiguability, polyuria and recent pain in her left knee. She denied any history of abdominal pain or haematemesis. Her appetite was poor and she had lost about half a stone in weight over the past 2 months. She was not on any drugs but occasionally took painkillers and antacid.

On examination she looked rather depressed and apathetic but was not confused. Her blood pressure was 160/90 pulse was 74/min regular. JVP not raised. Thyroid and lymph nodes were not palpable. There was no clubbing or obvious bony deformity but movements of the left knee were somewhat painful and limited with moderate joint effusion. Examination of the abdomen, respiratory and cardiovascular systems proved normal. She had loss of vibration sensation in both legs but tone and reflexes were normal.

The following were the results of various investigations:

Haemoglobin 12 g/dl
ESR 33 mm/1st hour
Urea 11 mmol/l
Electrolytes normal
Serum uric acid 300 μmol/l
Serum calcium 2.84 mmol/l
Phosphorus 0.8 mmol/l
Alkaline phosphatase 280 u/l
WBC 8.3 $\times$ 10^9/l
MCV 84 fl
Chest X-ray normal
Abdomen and pelvis X-ray normal
Left knee X-ray – Osteoarthritic changes with chondrocalcinosis
Calcium pyrophosphate crystals seen in joint fluid on aspiration

Questions

1 What is the most likely diagnosis?
2 What three other investigations will help this diagnosis?
3 Give five other causes of hypercalcaemia.

Answers to case 47

1 The finding of hypercalcaemia is obvious from the high serum calcium level with its effects, e.g. anorexia, vomiting, easy fatiguability, polyuria and general ill-health. Hypercalcaemia with low serum phosphorus and high serum alkaline phosphatase, bone pains with no abnormality on pelvis X-ray (no evidence of Paget's disease) and presence of chondrocalcinosis in the knee joint point towards the diagnosis of primary hyperparathyroidism.

2 (a) Estimation of urinary calcium over 24 h
(b) Prednisolone suppression test
(c) Radioimmunoassay for parathormone

3 (a) Malignancy with bony metastasis
(b) Multiple myeloma
(c) Vitamin D excess
(d) Thyrotoxicosis
(e) Paget's disease of bone

CASE 48

A 63-year-old lady was admitted with a 4-month history of deafness, poor mobility, falls, inability to cope on her own and generally getting slow and 'senile'. Her appetite had remained unchanged and though she could not be sure of weight gain or loss her daughter who visited her almost every week thought she had probably been putting on weight recently. There was no history of cough, expectoration, chest pain, palpitation, urinary or bowel symptoms.

She lived alone and had weekly home help and meals-on-wheels. She had not been out of her flat for the past 6 months.

On examination she was obese, pale and mildly confused. Her voice was gruff and rather hoarse. She had puffiness of both lower eyelids. Hair distribution was normal but her skin was somewhat dry and thickened. Blood pressure was 150/90 lying, 140/78 standing. No thyroid or lymph node enlargement. Apex beat was not easily palpable but she was in sinus rhythm with no heart murmur. Respiratory system and abdomen were normal. She had absent left ankle jerk with loss of sense of vibration but otherwise the neurological examination was unremarkable. On simple mental function testing she scored 8 out of 10.

The following were the results of various investigations:

Haemoglobin 10.9 g/dl
ESR 38 mm/1st hour
Electrolytes normal
WBC 7.4 × 10^9/l
MCV 84 fl
Blood urea 4.8 mmol/l
Blood glucose 4.9 mmol/l
Urine analysis – Protein ++; no sugar
MSU – *E. coli* growth

Questions

1 What is the most likely diagnosis?
2 What are the neuropsychiatric features of myxoedema?
3 What two investigations will confirm your diagnosis in this patient?

Answers to case 48

1 The most likely diagnosis in this elderly lady with a non-specific picture of declining mobility and general health, deafness, falls, slowness and senility, weight gain, mild confusion, puffiness of eyelids and dry skin is hypothyroidism. Hypothyroidism may present with atypical features in old age, and the diagnosis requires a high index of suspicion in these patients. In addition to myxoedema this lady has urinary tract infection as confirmed by urine culture report.

2 (a) Neurological: neuropathy, e.g. hearing loss; carpal tunnel syndrome; cerebellar syndrome
(b) Psychiatric: hallucinations; paranoid ideas; depression, attempted suicide; dementia (myxoedema madness)

3 (a) Serum T_3, T_4 and free thyroxine index
(b) TSH level

CASE 49

A 72-year-old lady went to see her doctor for a repeat prescription of her painkillers and antacids which she had been taking for her osteoarthritis and hiatus hernia for over 6 months. On routine check-up her blood pressure was found to be 210/110 mmHg. She denied having any chest pain, palpitation, cough, dyspnoea or oedema. Systemic examination was unremarkable but in view of her high blood pressure and risk of stroke, she was started on propranalol 80 mg three times a day with bendrofluazide 10 mg daily. Two days later she started experiencing giddiness, unsteadiness of legs, had two falls and became unable to look after herself. At this point she was admitted to the hospital for further investigation and rehabilitation.

On examination in the hospital her blood pressure was 150/90 sitting and 120/80 mmHg standing (she experienced dizziness on standing). There was no anaemia, clubbing or lymphadenopathy. She had an ejection systolic murmur at the apex and was in sinus rhythm. Chest and abdominal examination proved normal. Her fundi showed Grade I change of hypertension but there were no localizing neurological signs.

The following were the results of various investigations:

Haemoglobin 12.4 g/dl
ESR 30 mm/1st hour
Urea 8.3 mmol/l
Blood glucose 7.4 mmol/l
WBC $7.4 \times 10^9/l$
Sodium 135 mmol/l
Potassium 3.4 mmol/l
Chloride 96 mmol/l
Bicarbonate 27 mmol/l
ECG – Sinus rhythm, no infarction.
Urine analysis normal
Chest X-ray – Unfolding of aorta; no cardiomegaly; lung fields clear

Questions

1 What was the cause of her falls?
2 Under what circumstances would you not use antihypertensive drugs in people over the age of 75?
3 Give four side-effects of β-blockers in the elderly.

Answers to case 49

1 The sudden deterioration in her condition, including giddiness, unsteadiness of legs and falls, was almost certainly a result of rapid drop in blood pressure which resulted from the aggressive antihypertensive therapy (fairly high doses of propranolol and bendrofluazide).

A sudden reduction in blood pressure would be detrimental and can lead to various problems such as seen in this otherwise healthy lady. Reduction of blood pressure should always be achieved gently and slowly in the elderly.

2 Hypertension and its management in old age is a controversial area and the views differ. Practically no antihypertensive agent is free from side-effects and in some cases problems with drug therapy are far worse than the problem itself.
If a patient over 75 is asymptomatic and shows no signs of cardiac, renal or cerebral damage, no therapy is usually required.

3 (a) Increased risk of bronchospasm
(b) Precipitation of cardiac failure
(c) Cold hands and feet
(d) Confusion

CASE 50

A man of 70 with known angina, atrial fibrillation and mild diabetes was admitted with a 2-hour history of sudden severe central abdominal pain, vomiting and diarrhoea. There was no history of haematemesis or malaena. He had been taking occasional glyceryl trinitrate and digoxin 0.25 mg daily. His diabetes had been well controlled on a 150 g carbohydrate diet. On the day of this pain he had taken his usual food and tablets. There was no history of headaches, fits or faints.

On examination he was in pain, blood pressure 110/70. Pulse 84/min irregular, thyroid and lymph node not enlarged. No anaemia, clubbing or cyanosis. He was fibrillating with an apical rate of 90/min and had soft systolic apical murmur. Respiratory system was normal. In the abdomen he had diffused periumbilical tenderness but no guarding or rebound tenderness. Bowel sounds were faintly audible. Rectal examination was normal. Examination of nervous system was unremarkable.

The following were the results of various investigations:

Haemoglobin 13.4 g/dl
ESR 39 mm/1st hour
Blood glucose 7.9 mmol/l
Urea 12 mmol/l
Bicarbonate 24 mmol/l
WBC 13 × 10^9/l
Sodium 135 mmol/l
Potassium 3.6 mmol/l
Chloride 100 mmol/l
ECG – No acute changes of infarction
Chest X-ray – Heart size slightly enlarged; lung fields clear
X-ray abdomen – No fluid levels or air under the diaphragm

Questions

1 What is the most likely diagnosis?
2 How would you confirm your diagnosis?

Answers to case 50

1 The most likely diagnosis in this elderly man with ischaemic heart disease, atrial fibrillation and diabetes mellitus with sudden severe abdominal pain, vomiting, diarrhoea, low blood pressure, abdominal tenderness with faint bowel sounds and high white cell count with no acute myocardial infarction changes on the ECG is mesenteric artery occlusion, probably caused by thromboembolism. High index of suspicion in a patient with previous coronary artery disease and atrial fibrillation should always raise the possibility of such a complication.

2 The ultimate confirmation in such a patient with an acute abdomen (with no evidence of diabetic ketoacidosis) can be done only by emergency laparotomy. In fact on laparotomy this patient was found to have loops of gangrenous bowel.

CASE 51

Mrs A. W., a 68-year-old widow, was admitted to the hospital with a 6-week history of morning stiffness, pain and swelling of both hands and knees. She also complained of malaise, tiredness and difficulty in walking, cooking, dressing and making her own bed. Her own doctor had therefore arranged for a daily home help and meals-on-wheels 3 weeks ago.

On examination she looked unwell and anaemic. JVP was nil, blood pressure was 170/100, pulse 78/min regular, thyroid and lymph nodes were not enlarged. She had bilateral symmetrical swelling of her metacarpophalangeal and proximal interphalangeal joints with no subluxation. Both knee joints were also swollen with painful limitation of the movements. There were no subcutaneous nodules. Elbows, ankles, hips and shoulders were normal. She could walk only a few steps with the help of two nurses. Respiratory and cardiovascular systems and abdomen were normal. There were no neurological abnormalities.

Initial blood results were:

Haemoglobin 8.2 g/dl
ESR 85 mm/h
MCV 79 fl
WBC 8.3 × 10^9/l
Sodium 139 mmol/l
Potassium 3.6 mmol/l
Chloride 97 mmol/l
Urea 8.9 mmol/l

Questions

1 What is the most likely diagnosis?
2 What three further investigations will you ask for?
3 What are the ocular complications of rheumatoid arthritis?
4 Give six factors contributing to anaemia in rheumatoid arthritis.
5 What is palindromic rheumatism?

Answers to case 51

1 The most likely diagnosis is rheumatoid arthritis. Rheumatoid arthritis can commence at a late age in some patients. The female preponderance seen in younger patients tends to disappear in the elderly. Subcutaneous nodules and vasculitis are less commonly seen in patients with late-onset rheumatoid arthritis.

2 (a) X-rays of both hands and knees
(b) Rheumatoid factor
(c) Aspiration of joint fluid

3 (a) Episcleritis
(b) Keratoconjunctivitis sicca (Sjögren's syndrome)
(c) Corneal ulcer
(d) Uveitis
(e) Scleromalacia perforans

4 (a) Decreased ability to use iron
(b) Bleeding into the inflamed joints
(c) Gastrointestinal blood loss due to drugs
(d) Poor appetite and nutrition
(e) Bone marrow depression
(f) Haemolysis

5 Palindromic rheumatism is characterized by recurrent attacks of arthritis with periarticular inflammation but no residual joint deformity. The condition is distinctly different from rheumatoid arthritis but some of these patients have eventually been seen to develop rheumatoid arthritis.

CASE 52

A 48-year-old hospital administrator was referred to the medical outpatient department with a 3-month history of headaches, dizziness and fatigue. There was no particular pattern of the headaches and the patient thought that the headaches were as a result of pressure of extra work involved during the reorganization of his health district. There was no history of cough, expectoration, chest pain, palpitation, visual, urinary or bowel symptoms. He enjoyed good health until his present illness. He did not smoke or drink.

On examination he was comfortable. He had a ruddy complexion. His blood pressure was 165/110. Pulse was 74/min regular. JVP was not raised. There was no clubbing, oedema, thyroid or lymph node enlargement. Examination of cardiovascular and respiratory system proved normal. His spleen was 3 cm enlarged but there was no ascites or liver or kidney enlargement. Examination of central nervous system proved unremarkable.

The following were the results of various investigations:

Haemoglobin 18.3 g/dl
MCV 72 fl
WBC 24 × 10^9/l
Sodium 138 mmol/l
Potassium 3.9 mmol/l
Chloride 98 mmol/l
Bicarbonate 25 mmol/l
Blood glucose 4.3 mmol/l
Chest X-ray normal

Questions

1 What is the most likely diagnosis?
2 What three further investigations will you ask for?
3 Give four causes of secondary polycythaemia.
4 Give three measures which will help in the treatment of polycythaemia.

Answers to case 52

1 The most likely diagnosis in this 48-year-old gentleman with history of headaches, dizziness, fatigue, ruddy complexion, raised blood pressure, splenomegaly and raised haemoglobin, low MCV and raised white cell count is polycythaemia vera rubra.

2 (a) Estimation of red blood cell volume
(b) Bone marrow aspiration and biopsy
(c) Blood gases

3 (a) Pulmonary disease (chronic bronchitis, emphysema, pulmonary fibrosis)
(b) Cardiac conditions (ASD, VSD, dextroposition of aorta)
(c) Renal conditions (hydronephrosis, cystic disease and tumours)
(d) Tumours of liver, brain, prostate and breast, etc

4 (a) Venesection (if the haematocrit is over 55 per cent)
(b) Radioactive phosphorus therapy
(c) Chemotherapy with busulphan, chlorambucil or cyclophosphamide

CASE 53

K.M., a 69-year-old lady, was admitted with a 2-month history of confusion, unsteady gait and falls. During the week preceding her admission she had three falls and her husband, who was 66, found it difficult to cope with her failing health and old age. She had no loss of appetite or weight. Her daughter, who lived in the same street, visited her frequently and cooked for her parents about four times a week. There were no urinary or bowel symptoms.

On examination she was moderately confused. Blood pressure was 140/75, pulse 88/min regular. JVP was not raised and there was no oedema, thyroid or lymph node enlargement, clubbing or tremor. She looked slightly icteric. Respiratory system was normal. Her spleen was 2 cm enlarged but there was no hepatomegaly or ascites. She had an apical ejection systolic murmur, and was in sinus rhythm. Cranial nerves and fundi were normal. Power and tone were reduced in both legs with absent ankle jerk bilaterally, brisk knee reflexes with upgoing plantars bilaterally. Touch, pain and vibration sensations were impaired below the knee on both sides. Clinically there were no signs of fracture.

The following were the results of various investigations:

Haemoglobin 8.1 g/dl
Potassium 3.3 mmol/l
Sodium 140 mmol/l
Bicarbonate 25 mmol/l
Chloride 100 mmol/l
Bilirubin 23 μmol/l
Protein 63 g/l
Albumin 36 g/l
WBC 3.5×10^9/l; many hypersegmented neutrophils seen
ESR 39 mm/1st hour
MCV 112 fl
ECG – Some anterolateral ischaemia

Questions

1 What is the most likely diagnosis?
2 What three investigations will help the diagnosis?
3 How do you explain the presence of jaundice?
4 Name one other serious complication of pernicious anaemia.

Answers to case 53

1 The most likely diagnosis in this lady with confusion, unsteadiness of gait, falls, mild jaundice, splenomegaly, pyramidal and posterior column signs with low haemoglobin, and white cell count with hypersegmented neutrophils is B_{12} deficiency (probably pernicious anaemia) with subacute combined degeneration of the cord.

2 (a) Serum B_{12} and folate level
(b) Bone marrow aspiration
(c) Schilling test

3 Reticulocytosis with variable degree of haemolysis is commonly seen in many cases with pernicious anaemia. Mild jaundice in these patients is therefore a result of haemolysis.

4 Besides dementia (reversible) and subacute combined degeneration of the cord, carcinoma of the stomach is a recognized complication.

CASE 54

A 69-year-old lady was admitted with a 2-day history of severe right-sided abdominal pain and vomiting. There was no history of cough, expectoration or chest pain. The pain was constant in the right hypochondrium without any radiation. She had not been able to eat or drink much because of this illness.

On examination her temperature was 39°C, blood pressure 90/50, pulse 110/min regular. JVP was not raised. There was no anaemia, clubbing, thyroid or lymph node enlargement. She was dehydrated and mildly icteric and had rigors. There was marked guarding and tenderness in her right hypochondrium but no definite hepatomegaly. Spleen was not palpable and there was no ascites. Bowel sounds were audible. Respiratory, cardiovascular and neurological examination proved normal.

The following were the results of various investigations:

Haemoglobin 14.8 g/dl
Sodium 132 mmol/l
Potassium 3.9 mmol/l
Chloride 100 mmol/l
Bicarbonate 27 mmol/l
Blood urea 18 mmol/l
Blood glucose 8 mmol/l
WBC 24 × 10^9/l
ESR 73 mm/1st hour
Total protein 58 g/l
Albumin 28 g/l
Bilirubin 38 μmol/l
Gamma GT 118 u/l
Blood culture – *E. coli* growth sensitive to cephalosporin
Urine output in 24 h = 90 ml
Her condition improved with broad-spectrum antibiotics and intravenous fluids.

Questions

1 What is the most likely diagnosis?
2 Give four common organisms responsible for Gram-negative septicaemia in the elderly.
3 Give three common sources of septicaemia seen in the elderly.
4 Give four antibiotics which may be used against Gram-negative septicaemia

Answers to case 54

1 The most likely diagnosis in this elderly lady with right hypochondriac pain, vomiting, pyrexia rigors, low blood pressure, oliguria, abnormal gamma GT, raised white cell count and positive blood culture is septicaemia, probably caused by biliary tract disease with ascending cholangitis.

2 (a) **E. coli**
(b) **Strep. faecalis**
(c) **Pseudomonas aeruginosa**
(d) **B. proteus**

3 *(a)* ***Urinary tract infection with or without catheterization***
(b) ***Respiratory tract infection***
(c) ***Skin sores***

4 *(a)* ***Gentamycin***
(b) ***Carbenicillin***
(c) ***Collistin***
(d) ***Kanamycin***

CASE 55

Mrs P.K., a 58-year-old widow, was admitted with a 3-month history of generalized weakness, double vision and difficulty in swallowing, with weight loss. Her difficulty in swallowing and tiredness on chewing was getting progressively worse and she had recently started avoiding solid foods almost altogether and had lost half a stone in weight over the past 2 months. Double vision was not persistent but she had experienced it almost every day for past 4 weeks. On direct questioning she also admitted that she felt excessively tired and weak in her arms while combing her hair, and in fact had asked for a home help from the nearby social services office 2 weeks ago. There was no history of cough, expectoration, chest pain or palpitation. Her bowels were regular.

General physical examination was unremarkable with no swelling in the neck. She had bilateral ptosis, pupil size was normal on both sides with normal light and accommodation reflexes but she had diplopia on looking to the left. Fundi were normal. Motor, sensory systems and the reflexes were normal. The rest of the systemic examination was also normal.

The following were the results of various investigations:

Haemoglobin 13.2 g/dl
ESR 22 mm/1st hour
Sodium 138 mmol/l
Potassium 3.4 mmol/l
Chloride 96 mmol/l
Bicarbonate 25 mmol/l
WBC 9×9^{10}/l
Blood glucose 8.2 mmol/l
Blood urea 4.2 mmol/l
ECG normal

Questions

1 What is the most likely diagnosis?
2 Give three investigations to help the diagnosis.
3 Give one more investigation that you would like to include.
4 What is myasthenic syndrome?
5 Name three drugs that may help this patient.

Answers to case 55

1 The most likely diagnosis in this 58-year-old with diplopia, difficulty in chewing her food and combing her hair is myasthenia gravis.

2 (a) Tensilon test
(b) Electromyography
(c) Antibody screening test (anti acetylcholine receptor and antistriated muscle antibodies)

3 A chest X-ray (to look for thymus enlargement)

4 Myasthenic syndrome is characterized by weakness of muscles, as seen in true myasthenia gravis, but it is almost always associated with underlying malignancy. The syndrome is also known as Eaton–Lambert syndrome. Characteristic post-tetanic potentiation seen on electromyography helps to differentiate this syndrome from true myasthenia gravis.

5 (a) Neostigmine
(b) Pyridostigmine
(c) Corticosteroids

CASE 56

A man of 70 was admitted with a 4-month history of loss of weight of over 2 stone, poor appetite, generalized weakness and poor mobility. About 18 months ago he had his right eye enucleated. Apart from this enucleated eye he had always been fit and healthy. He lived in a ground-floor flat with his wife and had no social services. He did not smoke or drink. There was no history of cough, expectoration, chest pain, palpitation, urinary or bowel symptoms.

On examination he was pale and wasted. There was no clubbing, oedema or lymphadenopathy. Blood pressure was 140/70. Pulse 80/min regular. His skin was normal. There were no spider naevi, Dupuytren's contracture or palmar erythema. Examination of cardiovascular and respiratory system proved normal. His liver was 6 cm enlarged, hard, nodular, with an irregular surface and non-tender. Spleen was not palpable and there was no ascites. Rectal examination and proctoscopy proved normal. There were no significant findings in the nervous system apart from the right enucleated eye.

The following results were available:

Haemoglobin 8.4 g/dl
ESR 25 mm/1st hour
Sodium 134 mmol/l
Potassium 3.4 mmol/l
Chloride 100 mmol/l
Bicarbonate 24 mmol/l
Urea 8.9 mmol/l
Blood sugar 6.4 mmol/l
WBC 10 × 10^9/l
Platelet count normal

Questions

1 What is the most likely diagnosis?
2 What three investigations will you ask for?
3 Give four other sites commonly involved by malignant melanoma.

Answers to case 56

1 The most likely diagnosis in this elderly man with previous enucleation, poor appetite, significiant weight loss, cachexia and hepatomegaly is malignant melanoma with liver metastasis. Hard, irregular, nodular and non-tender liver is always suggestive of secondaries, and in this case the primary was more than likely in the enucleated eye.

2 (a) Liver function tests
(b) Abdominal ultrasound
(c) Liver biopsy

3 (a) Nails of fingers, toes
(b) Anus
(c) Nose, mouth
(d) Skin

CASE 57

A 69-year-old lady was admitted with a 6-week history of diarrhoea, weight loss of 1 stone, tiredness and lethargy. She denied having any abdominal pain or vomiting. The diarrhoea was in the form of three to five loose motions a day with no blood or mucus, but she had noticed at times that she had to flush the toilet repeatedly since the stools tended to float over the water.

She had always been fit and lived on her own in a second-floor council flat.

On examination she looked pale. JVP was not raised, no clubbing, lymphadenopathy or jaundice. Blood pressure was 145/85. Pulse 80/min. Thyroid not enlarged. In the abdomen there were no scars; liver spleen were not enlarged. Examination of respiratory, cardiovascular and nervous system proved normal.

The following investigation results were avilable:

Haemoglobin 8.5 g/dl
MCV 102 fl
Sodium 137 mmol/l
Potassium 3.1 mmol/l
Chloride 100 mmol/l
Bicarbonate 24 mmol/l
Urea 8 mmol/l
Blood glucose 7.4 mmol/l
Alkaline Phosphatase 80 u/l
WBC 9×10^9/l
ESR 23 mm/1st hour
Total protein 57 g/l
Albumin 32 g/l
Calcium 2.6 mmol/l
Phosphorus 1.1 mmol/l
Serum B_{12} 70 μg/l (normal 150–900 μg/l)
Serum folate 25 μg/l (normal 3–12 μg/l)
RBC folate 800 μg/l (normal 160–640 μg/l)
Faecal fat 10 g/24 h (normal less than 6 g/24 h)

Questions

1 What is the most likely diagnosis?
2 What is the cause of steatorrhoea in blind loop syndrome?
3 Give three investigations which can help in the diagnosis.

Answers to case 57

1 The diagnosis of malabsorption syndrome is clear from the history of diarrhoea, weight loss, low serum B_{12} and high faecal fat excretion. The finding of low serum B_{12} with a normal folate level further points towards the underlying cause being a blind loop syndrome resulting in stasis and bacterial colonization. Previous gastric or intestinal surgery, duodenal or jejunal diverticuli and diabetes mellitus are common causes for such a blind loop syndrome. In the elderly the blind loop syndrome may sometimes be seen without any obvious anatomical changes.

2 Bacterial overgrowth in the blind loop causes deconjugation of bile salts, which interferes with fat absorption. These deconjugated bile salts further act as irritants in the large gut and result in diarrhoea.

3 (a) Barium meal and follow-through

(b) ^{14}***C glycine cholate test***

(c) Duodenal/jejunal intubation and aspiration of contents for culture and bacterial count

CASE 58

A man of 72 was admitted with a 5-day history of malaise, generalized pains and bodyache, headaches and sore throat. For the past 2 days he had stopped eating and drinking, became confused and did not walk. He had no chest pain or palpitation. There were no urinary or bowel symptoms. He lived in an old people's home and because of his present illness the matron simply could not continue looking after him.

On examination his temperature was 38°C, his throat was congested and he was dehydrated. Cervical and axillary lymph nodes were palpable. There was no clubbing, anaemia, jaundice or oedema. He was confused and disorientated and thought the current year was 1942. Blood pressure was 160/95 and pulse was 92/min regular. Examination of cardiovascular and respiratory system proved normal. His spleen was 2 cm enlarged. Liver was not palpable and there was no ascites. Apart from confusion his neurological examination was normal.

The following results were available:

Haemoglobin 14.2 g/dl
ESR 38 mm/1st hour
Sodium 144 mmol/l
Potassium 3.2 mmol/l
Chloride 99 mmol/l
Bicarbonate 23 mmol/l
Urea 4.3 mmol/l
WBC 14 × 10^9/l
Polymorphs 38%
Lymphocytes 60%
Eosinophils 2%
Blood film – Many atypical lymphocytes seen
Chest X-ray normal
Blood sugar 7.8 mmol/l
Urine analysis normal

Questions

1 What is the most likely diagnosis?
2 What two investigations will confirm the diagnosis?
3 Give three serious complications of infectious mononucleosis.

Answers to case 58

1 The most likely diagnosis in this elderly man with flu-like illness, throat congestion, pyrexia, lymphadenopathy, splenomegaly and leucocytosis with high lympocytic count and atypical lymphocytes is infectious mononucleosis. Though infectious mononucleosis characteristically affects children and young adults, patients may be much older. In fact there have been a number of recent reports of elderly patients with infectious mononucleosis. Leukaemias and lymphomas should always be ruled out.

2 (a) Paul–Bunnell test for heterophil antibodies
(b) Antibody to Epstein–Barr virus (rising titres)

3 (a) Guillain–Barré syndrome
(b) Respiratory distress due to pharyngeal oedema
(c) Autoimmune haemolytic anaemia

CASE 59

A 23-year-old office clerk was admitted with a 2-day history of headache and sore throat. On the day of admission he woke up with chills, fever and painful joints. He had not been outside the United Kingdom for the past 6 years and had no history of blood transfusions or drug intake. He was unmarried and had enjoyed good health, but felt that he had been under undue pressure in his job in recent months. Four years ago he made an uneventful recovery from glandular fever. There were no other illnesses in the past. He smoked 20 cigarettes a day and enjoyed 4 to 5 pints of beer over most weekends.

On examination his temperature was 38°C. Blood pressure was 120/70. Pulse was 98/min regular. There was no anaemia, cyanosis, jaundice or oedema. Thyroid and lymph nodes were not enlarged. He had petechial rashes on his soft palate, both axillae and flanks. His throat was congested. His abdomen was soft. Liver was not enlarged but the spleen tip was palpable. Respiratory and central nervous systems were normal. He had neck rigidity and photophobia but the examination of fundi, cranial nerves, motor sensory system and reflexes was normal.

The following were the results of the initial investigations:

Haemoglobin 11 g/dl
White cell count 14.4 × 10^9/l
Platelets 250,000/mm^3
Prothrombin time 14 s
(Control 13 s)
Polymorphs 79%
Lymphocytes 18%
Basophils 2%
Eosinophils 1%
Blood urea 4.2 mmol/l
Blood glucose 6.9 mmol/l
Sodium 135 mmol/l
Potassium 4.7 mmol/l
Chloride 9.8 mmol/l
Bicarbonate 24 mmol/l
Serum creatinine 100 μmol/l
Urine examination – protein trace; 1–2WBC/HPF; no RBC
Chest X-ray – Heart size normal; no active lung lesion seen
ECG – Sinus tachycardia; heart rate 100/min
Paul–Bunnell test – Negative for infectious mononucleosis

Questions

1 What is the most likely diagnosis?
2 What four further investigations will you ask for?
3 Name three serious complications of meningococcal meningitis.
4 Name three antibiotics of choice for meningococcal meningitis.

Answers to case 59

1 The most likely diagnosis in this young patient with headaches; sore throat; pyrexia; petechial rashes in axillae, flanks and palate; pharyngitis; photophobia; neck stiffness; no lymphadenopathy; raised white cell count with polymorph leucocytosis; normal platelet count and negative Paul–Bunnell test is (meningococcal) meningitis.

2 (a) Lumbar puncture
(b) Blood culture
(c) Urine culture and sensitivity
(d) Throat swab culture

3 (a) Meningococcal septicaemia
(b) Disseminated intravascular coagulation
(c) Acute adrenal haemorrhage (Waterhouse-Friedrichsen syndrome)

4 (a) Penicillin G
(b) Ampicillin
(c) Sulphadiazine

CASE 60

A 65-year-old lady was admitted with a 3-month history of poor general health, aches and pains, shortness of breath on exertion, tiredness, weight loss of 6 pounds and poor appetite. She denied having chest pain, palpitation, cough or expectoration. There were no urinary or bowel symptoms. She lived alone and enjoyed her regular meals-on-wheels for the past 3 years, but not recently. In the past she had a successful partial gastrectomy for carcinoma of the stomach. She had not been taking any drugs.

On examination she was pale. Blood pressure 130/70, pulse 88/min regular. JVP not raised, no clubbing, thyroid or lymph node enlargement and oedema. Heart sounds were normal with an apical midsystolic murmur. Apex beat was in the fifth intercostal space in the midclavicular line. There was no hepatosplenomegaly or ascites or any other mass in the abdomen. Respiratory system was normal. Examination of cranial nerves, motor and sensory systems proved unremarkable.

The following were the results of various investigations:

Haemoglobin 8.2 g/dl
MCV 78 fl
Macrocyte +
Hypochromia +
Anisocytes +
Poikilocytes +
WBC 8.9 × 10^9/l
ESR 43 mm/1st hour
Blood glucose 5.6 mmol/l
Blood urea 11.3 mmol/l
Total protein 63 g/l
Albumin 32 g/l
Chest X-ray – Heart size slightly enlarged; unfolding of aorta; lung fields clear
Barium meal – Findings consistent with previous gastrectomy; no ulceration seen

Questions

1 What is the most likely diagnosis?
2 What further four investigations will you ask for?
3 How often should patients with previous gastrectomy be seen?

Answers to case 60

1 The most likely diagnosis in this 65-year-old lady with previous gastrectomy, carcinoma of stomach, general ill-health, aches and pains, shortness of breath, poor appetite, weight loss, anaemia with a mixed picture on peripheral blood film and a normal barium meal is probably anaemia (iron deficiency and/or B_{12} deficiency) with or without osteomalacia (aches and pains). Possibility of bony metastasis must also be borne in mind in a patient with previous malignancy.

2 (a) Serum calcium, phosphorus, alkaline phosphatase
(b) Serum B_{12}, folate, iron and iron-binding capacity
(c) Skeletal survey
(d) Bone scan

3 Patients should ideally be seen annually by their general practitioners to look for any evidence of recurrence of symptoms and features of deficiency of iron, B_{12} deficiency anaemia, osteoporosis or osteomalacia (with regular blood tests). Since there is a high incidence of these deficiency states, patients need to be followed up indefinitely.

CASE 61

A 72-year-old man living alone was admitted because of fall and inability to get up from the floor. His neighbours had found him on the floor in the afternoon and it was not quite certain how long he had been on the floor. History from the neighbour revealed that he had osteoarthritis of his knees, poor mobility, and had recently been started on some antidepressant tablets along with the painkillers. At home he had meals-on-wheels 5 days a week, home help once a week and walked with a Zimmer frame.

On examination he was confused and disorientated. Temperature was 33°C (axillary). Rectal temperature was 33.1°C. His skin was cold and clammy, with peripheral cyanosis. Blood pressure was 120/70, pulse 90/min regular. There was no clubbing or lymphadenopathy. He had marked osteoarthritis of the knees. Respiratory, cardiovascular and abdominal examination proved normal. Cranial nerves were intact and there were no localizing neurological signs.

The following were the results of various investigations:

Haemoglobin 14.2 g/dl
ESR 42 mm/1st hour
Urea 12 mmol/l
Blood glucose 8.8 mmol/l
Sodium 143 mmol/l
Potassium 3.1 mmol/l
Chloride 100 mmol/l
Bicarbonate 20 mmol/l
Chest X-ray — No lung lesion; heart size normal
ECG – Sinus rhythm with occasional ventricular ectopic; no infarction

Questions

1 What is the principal diagnosis?
2 Name four other drugs which commonly cause hypothermia in the elderly.
3 Why is rapid rewarming not recommended in the treatment of hypothermia?

Answers to case 61

1 The diagnosis in this elderly gentleman with low axillary and rectal temperature is obviously hypothermia. His fall may have been due to poor mobility with osteoarthritis. Further postural hypotension is a common side-effect of antidepressants in the elderly, and may have contributed to his fall. Confusion is consistent with the diagnosis of hypothermia but may also result from depression (pseudodementia) and antidepressant therapy. Hypothermia in the elderly usually results from a faulty temperature-regulatory mechanism, and may be coupled with one or more systemic illnesses or drug therapy such as with antidepressants.

2 (a) Phenothiazine tranquillizers
(b) Barbiturates
(c) Anticholinergic drugs
(d) Nitrazepam

3 Extensive cutaneous vasodilatation associated with rapid rewarming may result in falling arterial blood pressure and inadequate coronary perfusion. In some cases the vasodilatation allows cool blood to reach the body core, thus causing a further fall in central temperature.

CASE 62

S.S., a 72-year-old lady with kyphoscoliosis, osteoarthritis and mild Parkinsonism, was admitted with a 3-day history of generalized abdominal pain and vomiting for 24 hours before admission. She had no cough, expectoration, chest pain or palpitation. There were no urinary symptoms but she had no bowel action for the past 5 days.

She lived alone and had daily meals-on-wheels and a weekly visit by home help. She also attended a nearby day centre once a week.

On examination she was dehydrated. Blood pressure 140/60. Pulse was 88/min regular, no clubbing, anaemia, thyroid or lymph node enlargement. She was mildly confused and could not remember her own address. Abdomen was distended with some irregular mass in the left iliac fossa along the descending colon. Bowel sounds were faintly audible. Rectal examination confirmed the presence of a large amount of faeces. She had osteoarthritis of both knees, kyphoscoliosis, rest tremor and some rigidity in her limbs, but she could walk without any difficulty.

The following were the results of various investigations:

Haemoglobin 14 g/dl
Sodium 145 mmol/l
Potassium 4.6 mmol/l
Chloride 101 mmol/l
Bicarbonate 26 mmol/l
Blood glucose 9 mmol/l
Blood urea 12 mmol/l
WBC 8 × 10^9/l
Chest X-ray — No lung lesion; heart size normal
Abdomen X-ray — Fluid levels seen in the erect film

Questions

1 What is the diagnosis?
2 Give salient features of large bowel obstruction.

Answers to case 62

1 ***The most likely diagnosis in this lady with constipation, faecal impaction, abdominal pain and vomiting with fluid levels on erect abdominal films is intestinal obstruction, which has probably been caused by the faecal impaction. Constipation is comparatively uncommon but a recognized cause of large bowel obstruction, especially in the elderly.***

2 ***In contrast to small bowel obstruction, constipation lasting for days or weeks is the predominant feature followed by abdominal distension, especially in the flanks. Pain in large intestinal obstruction is usually more diffused, dull and continuous but may come in the form of colic, usually in the hypogastric region. It is not uncommon for vomiting to be delayed for 2–3 days. Plain abdominal X-rays may or may not show the fluid levels. The larger the number of fluid levels the nearer the obstruction is to the ileocaecal valve.***

CASE 63

A 62-year-old lady living alone was admitted for further investigation of her anaemia (haemoglobin 7.9 g/dl). She had a 3-month history of excessive weakness, fatigue, aches and pains. Her doctor thought that she was getting depressed and she had therefore been started on tricyclic antidepressants 9 weeks ago, but this had not helped her. Her appetite had not changed but she had lost 6 pounds in weight since being unwell. She denied having any urinary symptoms but admitted having a tendency towards constipation for at least 10 years. There was no history of cough, expectoration, palpitation, abdominal pain, headaches or visual disturbances. She had stopped smoking 15 years ago and enjoyed good health until her present illness.

On examination she was anaemic. Blood pressure was 160/90. Pulse was 84/min regular. There was no clubbing, jaundice, lymphadenopathy or thyroid enlargement. Her trachea was central and she had vesicular breathing all over her chest with no added sounds. Heart was in sinus rhythm with no murmurs. Her liver was 2 cm enlarged, soft and tender but she had no splenomegaly or ascites. Examination of the central nervous system proved normal.

The following were the results of various investigations:

Haemoglobin 7.9 g/dl
MCV 84 fl
ESR 119 mm/h
WBC 7.4 × 10^9/l
Sodium 140 mmol/l
Potassium 3.9 mmol/l
Chloride 98 mmol/l
Bicarbonate 24 mmol/l
Urea 11 mmol/l
Fasting blood glucose 4.9 mmol/l
Total protein 73 g/l
Albumin 24 g/l
Globulin 49 g/l
Urine analysis – Glucose nil, protein +, 2–4 WBCs/HPF
Chest X-ray – Heart size normal; lung fields clear

Questions

1 What is the most likely diagnosis?
2 What four further investigations will help your diagnosis?
3 List three drugs commonly used in chemotherapy of multiple myeloma.

Answers to case 63

1 The most likely diagnosis in this lady with non-specific complaints of fatigue, aches and pains, anaemia, high ESR, low serum albumin, raised globulins with no features of polymyalgia rheumatica (no headaches or visual disturbances) or diabetes mellitus (no glycosuria, normal blood glucose) is multiple myeloma. Carcinomatosis and lymphomas also need to be kept in mind, but are less likely in the absence of more specific features.

2 (a) Urine analysis for Bence Jones proteins
(b) Serum protein electrophoresis
(c) Skeletal survey
(d) Bone marrow aspiration and biopsy

3 (a) Corticosteroid
(b) Melphalan
(c) Cyclophosphamide

CASE 64

J.M., a 64-year-old retired British steelworker, was admitted with a 3-month history of progressively increasing weakness of his arms and legs with painful cramps and difficulty in walking. He had started using a walking stick for the past 2 months but during the past 2 weeks he could hardly stand without the help of his wife.

On examination he was mentally alert, blood pressure was 160/80 and pulse was 80/min regular. Thyroid and lymph nodes were not enlarged and there was no clubbing or anaemia. Peripheral pulses were palpable. Examination of cardiovascular and respiratory systems and abdomen proved normal. Cranial nerves were normal. There was marked bilateral wasting and weakness of shoulder girdle muscles bilaterally with winging of the scapulae. He had claw hand deformity in the left hand. There was marked fasciculation over both upper arms and thighs. There was some wasting and weakness of muscles of both lower limbs. Tendon reflexes were depressed in the upper limbs but brisk in lower limbs with upgoing plantars. There was no sensory impairment.

Initial investigation results were as follows:

Haemoglobin 14.2 g/dl
Serum B_{12} and folate normal
MCV 89 fl
WBC 9×10^9/l
ESR 40 mm/h
Urea and electrolytes normal
Chest X-ray normal
ECG normal
Blood sugar 6 mmol/l

Questions

1 What is the most likely diagnosis?
2 What four investigations will you ask for?
3 What is the prognosis of this condition?

Answers to case 64

1 ***The most likely diagnosis in this 64-year-old man with gradually increasing weakness and wasting of his arms and legs with cramps, claw hand deformity, winging of scapulae, fasciculations, depressed tendon reflexes in upper limbs (lower motor neurone), and increased reflexes in lower limbs (upper motor neurone) with no sensory impairment is motor neurone disease.***

2 ***(a) Electromyography***
(b) Nerve conduction studies
(c) Muscle biopsy
(d) Serum creatine phosphakinase activity

3 ***Unfortunately the prognosis in most cases is poor, with death due to respiratory failure and bronchopneumonia within 2–3 years after the onset of symptoms.***

CASE 65

A 62-year-old widow was admitted with a history of increasing shortness of breath, tiredness and poor appetite for the past 4 months. She had also lost half a stone in weight during this period. Her previous medical illness included a fall with Colles fracture 2 years ago, osteoarthritis and Parkinsonism, for which she was taking regular paracetamol and L-dopa for the past year. Six months ago she contracted a urinary tract infection which settled with co-trimoxazole treatment. She lived alone and attended the nearby day centre twice weekly.

On examination she was dyspnoeic and moderately anaemic. Blood pressure was 170/90, pulse was 110/min regular. JVP was not raised, clubbing was absent with no thyroid enlargement. There was no palmar erythema or spider naevi. Lymph nodes were not palpable. Heart was in sinus rhythm with a soft systolic apical murmur. Respiratory system was normal. Liver was 3 cm enlarged, firm, smooth and non-tender with no bruit. The spleen was 9 cm enlarged. There was no ascites. Neurological examination was essentially normal.

Her initial blood tests were reported as follows:

Haemoglobin 8.6 g/dl
ESR 53 mm/1st hour
Urea 8.4 mmol/l
Sodium 143 mmol/l
Potassium 3.3 mmol/l
Chloride 97 mmol/l
Bilirubin 13 μmol/l
Total platelet count normal
WBC 89 $\times$ 10^9/l
Uric acid 780 μmol/l

Questions

1 What is the most likely diagnosis?
2 What three further investigations can help the diagnosis?
3 What is the role of splenectomy in chronic myeloid leukaemia?
4 What is the prognosis of chronic myeloid leukaemia in the elderly?

Answers to case 65

1 The most likely diagnosis in this patient with anaemia, massive splenomegaly and mildly enlarged liver is either chronic myeloid leukaemia (CML) or myelofibrosis.

2 (a) Bone marrow aspiration and biopsy
(b) Philadelphia chromosome
(c) Neutrophil alkaline phosphatase (reduced in CML)

3 Splenectomy is not indicated in patients with chronic myeloid leukaemia. Only rare patients with constant dragging pain due to massive splenomegaly may be helped by splenectomy.

4 The median survival time is 2–3 years in the elderly; this is a year or two less than in younger adults.

CASE 66

A 62-year-old lady was admitted with a 2-month history of progressive shortness of breath on exertion, tiredness, poor appetite and loss of weight of 6 pounds. She denied having any cough, expectoration or haemoptysis. There were no urinary or bowel symptoms and she was not taking any drugs.

She lived alone in a ground-floor flat and had a home help twice a week. Six months ago she had enjoyed 2 weeks holiday with her sister in Scotland.

On examination she was dyspnoeic. JVP was not raised, there was no anaemia, clubbing, cyanosis, oedema or lymphadenopathy. Trachea was central. Over her right base posteriorly she had dullness on percussion with absent breath sounds and diminished vocal fremitus and resonance. Apex beat was in the fourth intercostal space well inside the midclavicular line. She had no heart murmurs. Examination of abdomen and central nervous system proved normal.

The following were the results of various investigations:

Haemoglobin 11.6 g/dl
ESR 68 mm/1st hour
Sodium 137 mmol/l
Potassium 3.3 mmol/l
Bicarbonate 24 mmol/l
WBC 8 × 10^9/l
Blood urea 11 mmol/l
Blood sugar 18.9 mmol/l
Chest X-ray – Heart size normal; right pleural effusion
ECG normal

Questions

1 What is the most likely diagnosis?
2 What are three other common causes of pleural effusion in the elderly?
3 What three investigations will you ask for in this patient?
4 Give three conditions associated with transudative pleural effusion.

Answers to case 66

1 It is obvious from the physical examination and investigations that she has right pleural effusion and diabetes mellitus (high blood glucose). Tuberculosis often has an atypical presentation in the elderly, and the absence of a cough or expectoration should not therefore be surprising. Further, diabetic patients are prone to conditions like tuberculosis; hence tubercular pleural effusion is most likely to be the case in this elderly lady.

2 (a) Heart failure
(b) Malignancy
(c) Pneumonia

3 (a) Aspiration of pleural fluid for cytology; AFB and biochemistry
(b) Sputum for AFB; malignant cells
(c) Pleural biopsy

4 (a) Heart failure
(b) Nephrotic syndrome
(c) Meig's syndrome

CASE 67

Mrs P.L., a 64-year-old lady, was admitted on New Year's Eve with a 4-day history of almost continuous severe backache, worse on stooping – e.g. making her own bed. There was no radiation of pain, and coughing and sneezing did not make much difference to the pain. She denied any history of lifting heavy weight or trauma. Her own doctor thought she had probably been overdoing things over Christmas and advised bed rest, told her to take things easy, and started her on paracetamol tablets as required. This treatment did not help her much as she had restless nights and had pain on turning position in the bed for the past 2 nights.

On examination she appeared to be in pain. There was no anaemia, clubbing or lymphadenopathy. JVP was not raised. She had bilateral osteoarthritis of her knees, kyphoscoliosis and some tenderness over her T_{12}–L_1 region on the back. Straight leg raising test was normal. Examination of abdomen, respiratory and cardiovascular systems proved normal. Cranial nerves were intact, motor and sensory system normal. She had absent left ankle jerk with loss of sense of vibration. All other tendon reflexes were normal with bilateral downgoing plantars.

The following were the results of various investigations:

Haemoglobin 13.4 g/dl
ESR 29 mm/1st hour
Sodium 137 mmol/l
Potassium 4.1 mmol/l
Chloride 97 mmol/l
Bicarbonate 25 mmol/l
WBC 8.7 × 10^9/l
Blood urea 9.2 mmol/l
Blood glucose 6.3 mmol/l
Calcium 2.25 mmol/l
Phosphorus 1.01 mmol/l
Alkaline phosphatase 70 u/l
X-ray dorsolumbar spine – Crush fracture of L_{1-2} vertebrae with increased translucency of bones

Questions

1 What is the most likely diagnosis?
2 What two further investigations will you ask for?
3 Why did rest and immobilization fail to help this patient?
4 What are the endocrinal causes of osteoporosis?

Answers to case 67

1 The most likely diagnosis in this elderly lady with sudden severe backache made worse by movements of her back with no radiation, unaffected by milder analgesics, no anaemia, kyphoscoliosis, tenderness over T_{12}–L_1 region, normal straight leg raising test, normal serum calcium, phosphorus and alkaline phosphatase and crush fracture of L_1–$_2$ vertebrae with increased bony translucency is osteoporosis. The absence of vibration sense and ankle jerk is not uncommon in healthy elderly people.

2 (a) Immunoglobulin electrophoresis (to rule out multiple myeloma)
(b) Trephine biopsy of the bones for histological confirmation of the diagnosis

3 ***Rest and immobilization contribute to further loss of bone density and are therefore not advisable. Patients must always be encouraged to maintain their mobility with adequate pain control.***

4 ***(a) Hyperthyroidism***
(b) Cushing's syndrome
(c) Acromegaly
(d) Diabetes mellitus

CASE 68

P.K., a 47-year-old senior civil servant, was admitted with history of confusion, nausea, vomiting and jaundice for 2 weeks. He had not been taking any drugs recently but had received a blood transfusion 3 years ago after gastrectomy. Also postoperatively he had to be sedated with phenothiazine for 2 nights. He had a 20-year history of heavy drinking and had recently been drinking up to one bottle of whisky a day since the death of his wife 10 months ago. He had recently moved into a flat in the west end of London. His only daughter lived in Australia and her last visit was 5 years ago.

On examination he looked thin and emaciated. He was confused and moderately jaundiced and had scratch marks on both his legs and abdomen. There was no clubbing or lympadenopathy. He had five spider naevi on his face, neck and upper chest, palmar erythema more marked on the left palm and bilateral Dupuytren's contracture. Blood pressure was 170/110. Pulse was 100/min regular. His heart was in sinus rhythm and he had no heart murmurs.

In the abdomen his liver was 4 cm enlarged, tender and smooth with a regular edge. There was no splenomegaly or ascites.

His initial investigations were reported as:

Haemoglobin 13 g/dl
WBC 11 × 10^9/l
Sodium 136 mmol/l
Potassium 3.1 mmol/l
Chloride 95 mmol/l
Urea 4 mmol/l
MCV 110 fl
Bilirubin 88 μmol/l
ALT 200 u/l
AST 320 u/l
Alkaline phosphatase 210 u/l

Questions

1 What is the most likely diagnosis?
2 What three further investigations will you ask for?
3 What is the significance of scratch marks?
4 Could this jaundice be the result of chlorpromazine taken 3 years ago.
5 Name four other commonly used drugs which may cause jaundice.

Answers to case 68

1 The most likely diagnosis in this 47-year-old patient with history of heavy drinking and signs of liver cell failure (i.e. spider naevi, palmar erythema, Dupuytren's contracture and hepatomegaly) is acute alcoholic hepatitis.

2 (a) Australia antigen
(b) Barium swallow to look for oesophageal varices
(c) Liver biopsy after checking prothrombin time

3 Jaundice in acute alcoholic cirrhosis may have the features of obstructive rather than hepatocellular jaundice, and will result in excessive circulating bile salts, which is thought to be the cause of pruritus and scratching.

4 *No, since the drug was taken so long ago this is unlikely to be the case. Jaundice caused by chlorpromazine is seen usually within days to weeks of initial drug exposure.*

5 (a) *Antidepressants*
(b) *Benzodiazepines such as diazepam*
(c) *Oral hypoglycaemic agents such as chlorpropamide*
(d) *Anabolic hormones such as testosterone*

CASE 69

A lady of 72 was admitted with acute on chronic bronchitis. The day after her admission she woke up with severe pain and swelling of her right big toe. There was no clear history of trauma but she did admit to having a fall at home the day before her admission. She could remember having similar pain in her right big toe about 4 years ago, which had settled within a week with no treatment. The only medication that she had been taking was salbutamol tablets which she took whenever she felt a bit chesty.

On examination her blood pressure was 190/100, pulse 82/min regular. JVP was not raised and thyroid was not enlarged. Her right big toe was red, hot and tender. Her peripheral pulses, except for the right dorsalis pedis artery, were palpable. Cardiovascular and abdominal examination was normal. In the respiratory system she had widespread rhonchi with bilateral basal crepitations. The right ankle jerk was absent but the rest of the neurological examination was normal.

The following results of investigations were available:

Haemoglobin 12.9 g/dl
ESR 40 mm/h
WBC 9 × 10^9/l
Sodium 136 mmol/l
Potassium 3.6 mmol/l
Chloride 94 mmol/l
Bicarbonate 27 mmol/l
Blood urea 8.9 mmol/l
Blood glucose 5.4 mmol/l
Chest X-ray–Changes consistent with chronic bronchitis and emphysema: no pneumothorax

Questions

1 What is the most likely diagnosis, and why?
2 What are two other possibilities you might consider?
3 What three investigations would you request?
4 Name two helpful drugs for acute gouty attacks.

Answers to case 69

1 The most likely diagnosis is an acute gouty attack affecting her right metatarsophalangeal joint. Most probably she had a similar acute gouty attack about 4 years ago which settled without any treatment.

2 (a) Local trauma. Although there is a history of fall in this patient no clear history of local trauma is available
(b) Infective arthritis

3 (a) Serum uric acid
(b) X-ray of her right foot
(c) Aspiration of the joint

4 (a) Colchicine
(b) Indomethacin

CASE 70

A 63-year-old lady living alone was admitted with a 2-week history of difficulty in walking and a fall on the day of her admission. There was no history of loss of consciousness, palpitation or chest pain. She denied having dizzy spells but on direct questioning admitted having frequent left-sided headaches for the past 5 weeks. There was no history of vomiting, loss of appetite or weight. She had been known to suffer with depression 2 years ago, and was taking amytryptiline 50 mg every night.

On examination she was found to be moderately confused and apathetic. She was not anaemic, cyanosed or jaundiced. There was no clubbing, thyroid or lymph node enlargement. Blood pressure was 160/100. Pulse was 50/min regular. She had a soft systolic apical murmur. Examination of abdomen and respiratory system proved normal. Cranial nerves were normal but on fundus examination she was noticed to have some blurring of the disc margins on both sides. She had upper motor neurone signs of right-sided weakness with increased reflexes and upgoing right plantar. Over the next 24 hours her right-sided weakness deteriorated and she became much more drowsy. After an urgent CT brain scan she was started on intravenous dexamethasone but died suddenly after 24 hours.

Questions

1 What is the most likely diagnosis?
2 What is the probable cause of her death?
3 What is the explanation for her slow pulse rate?
4 What is the role of the steroid in the treatment of brain tumour?

Answers to case 70

1 Brain tumour is the most likely diagnosis in this patient. A previous history of depression or any other mental illness should not make one forget the possibility of an organic lesion. Slow onset of the symptoms, progressive depression in the mental status, and weakness of the limbs all point towards the strong possibility of intracranial space-occupying lesion. In fact the diagnosis of brain tumour was confirmed on the CT scan in this patient.

2 Sudden haemorrhage in the brain tumour is the most likely explanation for her rapid deterioration and death.

3 Brain tumour causing raised intracranial pressure is the most likely cause for her bradycardia.

4 Dexamethasone was given to this patient in an effort to reduce the cerebral oedema. The use of dexamethasone, however, remains controversial.

CASE 71

Mrs S., a 72-year-old lady with Parkinsonsim, had been taking L-dopa for over 3 years. Her general practitioner was called to see her at home over the weekend since she had started falling recently. The general practitioner had failed to find any significant change in her Parkinsonism and she was sent to the hospital for further assessment and rehabilitation.

On examination in the hospital she was found to be mentally alert. She had some features of Parkinsonism, i.e. she had tremor at rest, but there was no rigidity. She had an expressionless face but her gait was steady. Examination of cardiovascular and respiratory systems proved normal. Later during the day, as she was walking towards the day room, she was reported by the nursing staff to be completely immobile as if her feet had frozen on the floor after walking only a few steps. She had to sit for a few minutes in the chair, but surprisingly could walk well later on. These 'funny spells' were seen to recur next day once again. Physical examination otherwise remained unremarkable. Her haemoglobin full blood count ESR and urea and electrolytes were all reported as normal.

Questions

1 What is the possible explanation for her sudden change during the day?
2 Does this patient require an increase in her L-dopa doses?
3 How can a physician avoid side-effects such as on–off phenomenon altogether?

Answers to case 71

1 ***This lady with Parkinsonism, on L-dopa therapy, has probably been having on–off phenomenon, being unable to move at times. On–off attacks may recur several times a day in the same patient. The aetiology of the on–off phenomenon remains far from clear.***

2 ***No. On the contrary the dose of L-dopa probably needs to be reduced.***

3 ***By avoiding the use of L-dopa in most mild cases. In patients with milder forms of Parkinsonism symptoms may be effectively controlled simply by using anticholinergic agents, e.g. benzhexol (Artane) or orphenadrine (Disipal) and amantadine (Symmetrel). Bromocriptine has recently been used for Parkinsonism and is certainly a good alternative in patients where side-effects of L-dopa such as on–off phenomenon limit its effectiveness. Bromocriptine can be safely used in combination with L-dopa.***

CASE 72

A 64-year-old lady was admitted with a 2-day history of malaena. She was known to have osteoarthritis of her right hip and knee, and had been taking various painkillers for the past 4 years. Because of her increasing pain and decreasing mobility she was given a supply of Naprosyn tablets only a week ago. There was no history of vomiting or haematemesis but on direct questioning she did admit to have indigestion for the past 8 months with occasional difficulty in swallowing. There was no history of loss of appetite or weight. She had had a tendency towards constipation for the past 15 years and had been taking some laxatives about once a week for the past 5 years.

On examination she was found to be anaemic, There was no jaundice, clubbing, oedema, thyroid or lymphadenopathy. Blood pressure was 110/60. Pulse was 88/min regular. She was tender over her epigastrium but there was no mass, or hepatosplenomegaly. Examination of respiratory, cardiovascular and neurological system was normal.

The following were the results of various initial investigations:

Haemoglobin 8.6 g/dl
MCV 73 fl
Urea 12.7 mmol/l
Sodium 139 mmol/l
Potassium 3.4 mmol/l
Chloride 96 mmol/l
Bicarbonate 24 mmol/l
Chest X-ray normal
ECG normal

Questions

1 What is the most likely cause of her malaena?
2 What are the indications of blood transfusion in patients with gastrointestinal bleeding?
3 What anti-inflammatory agent would you choose for this patient?

Answers to case 72

1 Bleeding gastric ulcer is the most likely cause of gastrointestinal bleed in this patient. Virtually all non-steroidal anti-inflammatory agents are capable of causing gastrointestinal bleed in both young and elderly patients. In fact this patient was found on endoscopy to have an acute gastric erosion.

2 The decision to transfuse is always made on clinical grounds. In most cases one or more of the following findings indicate a need for blood transfusion:
(a) A pulse rate of over 100/min
(b) Systolic blood pressure of less than 100.
(c) Haemoglobin less than 10 g/dl

3 In view of her dyspepsia and gastrointestinal bleed none of the presently available anti-inflammatory agents can be considered safe for this patient. Pain from her osteoarthritis should preferably be controlled by regular analgesics such as paracetamol.

CASE 73

A 24-year-old unmarried piano teacher was referred to the medical out-patient department with a 3-month history of easy bruising and tiredness. She had no history of cough, expectoration, haemoptysis, chest or joint pain. Her appetite was good and she had not lost any weight. There were no urinary or bowel symptoms. She had started menstruating at the age of 15, her periods were regular but for the past 6 months she had noticed that her bleeding was excessive and lasted for 4–5 days. She was not taking any pills. She smoked 10–15 cigarettes a day and took alcohol only occasionally.

On examination she looked pale. Blood pressure was 120/70. Pulse was 80/min regular. There was no clubbing, cyanosis, jaundice, oedema, thyroid or lymph node enlargement. There were petechial haemorrhages over both her legs and thighs. Examination of locomotor system, cardiovascular, respiratory and central nervous systems proved unremarkable. Her abdomen was soft and there was no hepatosplenomegaly.

The results of the initial investigations were as follows:

Haemoglobin 11.2 g/dl
MCV 78 fl
WBC 8 × 10^9/l
Platelet count 38,000/mm^3
Prothrombin time 14 s
(Control 13 s)
Sodium 139 mmol/l
Potassium 4.1 mmol/l
Chloride 100 mmol/l
Bicarbonate 24 mmol/l
Blood glucose (random) 5.3 mmol/l
Blood urea 4.2 mmol/l
Chest X-ray normal
Capillary fragility test positive

Questions

1 What is the most likely diagnosis?
2 What three further investigations will you ask for?
3 How do you treat idiopathic thrombocytopenic purpura?

Answers to case 73

1 The most likely diagnosis in this young lady with easy bruising, purpuric spots, menorrhagia, no splenomegaly, low platelet count, normal prothrombin time and blood urea and positive capillary fragility test is thrombocytopenic purpura. There are many causes of thrombocytopenia, e.g. marrow infiltration, drug therapy and decreased platelet survival. Idiopathic thrombocytopenic purpura is a likely diagnosis in this patient in the absence of the history of drug intake, normal blood urea and a good general health with no other significant physical findings. In most cases idiopathic thrombocytopenic purpura is a diagnosis of clinical exclusion.

2 (a) Bleeding and clotting time
(b) Platelet autoantibodies
(c) Bone marrow aspiration and biopsy

3 (a) Medical therapy with high-dose steroids
(b) Splenectomy in cases of failure of medical therapy

CASE 74

A 64-year-old lady was admitted with history of frequent falls for the past 6 weeks. Three weeks ago she was seen in the accident and emergency department after a fall at home. The casualty officer had sent her home after X-ray of her chest and pelvis with a letter to her general practitioner stating 'no bony injury'. She denied having any significant illnesses in the past.

On examination she was found to be moderately confused. There was no anaemia, cyanosis, jaundice, oedema, clubbing, thyroid or lymph node enlargement. She had some bruising over her knees and right temporal region. Examination of respiratory and cardiovascular systems proved normal. There were signs of upper motor neurone paralysis affecting her left side with increased tone and an upgoing plantar.

Since she was unable to give a detailed account of her falls the admitting doctor decided to interview a visiting neighbour who described that the elderly lady was getting progressively confused over the past 9 months and had been drinking six to eight Guinnesses a day for at least the past 10 years, since she had known her. Two days after her admission the patient was reported by the nursing staff to be in a variable mood, being cheerful and alert at times and quite confused and apathetic on other occasions. A more thorough neurological examination on the next morning confirmed the presence of left-sided weakness with upper motor neurone signs. She was also noted to have a dilated pupil on the right side but there was no loss of light or accommodation reflexes. Fundi were normal.

Questions

1 What is the most likely diagnosis?
2 What three further investigations will you ask for?
3 Give three possible causes of confusion in this lady?

Answers to case 74

1 The most likely diagnosis in this elderly lady with history of alcoholism, confusion, frequent falls, bruising over her right temporal region, fluctuation in the level of her consciousness, a dilated right pupil and left-sided weakness is subdural haematoma.

2 (a) Skull X-ray
(b) CT brain scan
(c) Liver function test

3 (a) Subdural haematoma
(b) Alcoholism
(c) Senile dementia

CASE 75

A 62-year-old lady was admitted with sudden right-sided weakness, visual loss and confusion. There was no history of chest pain, palpitation, cough, expectoration, bowel or urinary symptoms. She had been previously admitted with two transient ischaemic attacks but was discharged with no medication.

On examination she was moderately confused. JVP was not raised. There was no anaemia, jaundice, cyanosis, clubbing, thyroid or lymph node enlargement. Blood pressure was 150/95. Pulse was 78/min regular. She had no carotid bruits. Examination of cardiovascular and respiratory systems and abdomen proved normal. There was complete loss of visual acuity but eye movements were normal. Fundi were normal with no blurring of the disc margins. Pupillary reflexes were normal as well. Examination of the cranial nerves proved unremarkable. She had signs of upper motor neurone paralysis on the right side with increased tone, brisk reflexes and upgoing right plantar.

Questions

1 What is the most likely diagnosis?
2 How do you explain the presence of normal pupillary reflexes?
3 What is the single most important differential diagnosis?
4 What is the single most useful investigation you can ask for?

Answers to case 75

1 The most likely diagnosis in this lady with right-sided weakness, loss of vision and confusion with previous history of transient ischaemic attacks is cerebrovascular accident involving posterior cerebral arteries resulting in cortical damage and blindness.

2 In cases of cortical blindness the afferent and efferent course of the light and accommodation reflexes does not involve the postcerebral cortex and therefore the pupillary reflexes normally remain unaffected.

3 The most important differential diagnosis is hysterical blindness. However in an otherwise healthy elderly lady with no previous pyschiatric history this is unlikely. Hysteria may occasionally present both with sudden blindness and hemiplegia.

4 CT brain scan for localization of area of cerebral infarct.

CASE 76

A 73-year-old man with Parkinsonism was started on levodopa increasing to 250 mg three times a day. Over the next few days his rigidity and bradykinesia improved considerably but unfortunately he started getting increasing tremor of his hands. He became agitated and depressed and complained of continuing sickness. To control these symptoms effectively he was given metoclopramide (Maxolon) and diazepam. The sickness and agitational status improved but he started losing his mobility and independence in dressing and undressing. Nursing staff reported next day that he had been feeling rather low, complained of weakness and had asked for a particular tonic which had helped him 3 years ago. He was given some multivitamin tablets. However, his general condition deteriorated over the next few days and all that he wanted was to be left alone in bed.

The following were the results of various investigations at this stage:

Haemoglobin 13 g/dl
ESR 34 mm
WBC 9×9^{10}/l
Sodium 139 mmol/l
Potassium 3.4 mmol/l
Chloride 102 mmol/l
Bicarbonate 25 mmol/l
Blood glucose 7.1 mmol/l
Blood urea 9.9 mmol/l
Chest X-ray normal
ECG – Sinus rhythm, with occasional ventricular ectopic

Questions

1 Why did the patient get increasing tremor on levodopa therapy?
2 Why did the patient get worse on metoclopramide and diazepam?
3 Name three other drugs which should be avoided, or used with care, in a patient on levodopa.

Answers to case 76

1 Levodopa is useful in relieving many of the symptoms of Parkinsonism, particularly rigidity and bradykinesia. In many cases it helps in controlling tremor but occasionally the tremor may get worse.

2 Metoclopramide is a dopamine antagonist and thus reduces the effect of levodopa. Diazepam and pyridoxine (in multivitamin tablets) are also known to have adverse drug interactions with levodopa.

3 (a) Phenothiazine
(b) MAO inhibitor
(c) Phenytoin

CASE 77

Mrs B.D., a 64-year-old lady living alone, was admitted because of self-neglect, inability to look after herself and 'dementia'. Since the death of her husband 4 months ago she had stopped going to the nearby bingo club. On one occasion 3 weeks ago she thought she could hear the voice of her dead husband. There was no history of cough, expectoration, chest pain, palpitation, urinary or bowel symptoms. Her appetite had declined recently and she had lost 5 pounds in weight in the past 3 months. There was no previous history of any significant illness.

On examination she appeared depressed and apathetic. She denied having suicidal ideas but did think that life was not worth living any more. She was slow and inattentive but was not confused. Blood pressure was 140/85 and pulse was 78/min regular. There was no anaemia, cyanosis, jaundice, oedema, thyroid or lymph node enlargement. Examination of respiratory system, cardiovascular system and abdomen proved normal. There were no focal neurological signs.

The following were the results of various investigations:

Haemoglobin 12.8 g/dl
MCV 78 fl
WBC 8.2×10^9/l
ESR 38 mm/h
Sodium 139 mmol/l
Potassium 3.4 mmol/l
Chloride 96 mmol/l
Bicarbonate 24 mmol/l
Urea 7.9 mmol/l
Random blood glucose 6.2 mmol/l
Chest X-ray normal
ECG normal

Questions

1 What is the most likely diagnosis?
2 What are the common side-effects of tricyclic antidepressant drugs?
3 Is the presence of auditory hallucination against the diagnosis of depression (pseudodementia)?

Answers to case 77

1 The most likely diagnosis in this 64-year-old lady with an acute onset of illness, starting soon after a stressful event, i.e. the death of her husband, is depression. Depression causing pseudodementia must be differentiated from true dementia, which has a slow and insiduous onset and is usually not preceded by a stressful event. In fact this lady made a good recovery a few weeks after she was started on tricyclic antidepressants.

2 (a) Anticholinergic side-effects such as dry mouth, blurring of vision, constipation and urinary retention
(b) Postural hypotension
(c) Cardiac arrhythmias and heart blocks

3 No, though various types of hallucinations are far more common in dementia, occasionally auditory hallucinations may occur in patients with depression.

CASE 78

A 76-year-old lady was admitted with a 3-month history of right-sided facial pain affecting the area of her right cheek and lower eyelid. The pain was described as an electric shock, and lasted only for a few seconds. During the past 3 weeks she had been getting these pains up to five to six times a day, and was getting afraid even to wash her face in the morning. There was no history of cough, expectoration, chest pain, palpitation, headaches, blurring of vision, urinary or bowel symptoms. The pain did not wake her during night-time. The only significant past history was of shingles 20 years ago.

On examination she was mentally alert. Blood pressure was 160/100, pulse 90/min regular. There was no clubbing or lymphadenopathy. Respiratory and cardiovascular systems were normal. Cranial nerves were intact with no motor or sensory impairment, fundi were normal and her reflexes were equal on both sides.

Initial results of the investigations were as follows:

Haemoglobin 12.7 g/dl
ESR 31 mm/1st hour
Urea and electrolytes normal
Chest X-ray normal

Questions

1 What is the most likely diagnosis?
2 Is there any significance of past history of shingles?
3 What is the most effective drug therapy for trigeminal neuralgia?

Answers to case 78

1 The most likely diagnosis in this elderly lady with attacks of sharp, short-lived facial pain with no localizing neurological signs is trigeminal neuralgia.

2 Since she has remained free of pain for 20 years this is certainly not a case of post-herpetic neuralgia. In cases with post-herpetic neuralgia patients may continue with severe sharp pains in the area of scarring and may become extremely depressed.

3 Carbamazepine is the most effective therapy for trigeminal neuralgia and is seen to be helpful in the majority of these patients.

CASE 79

A 68-year-old retired headmaster was admitted with an 18-hour history of polyuria, excessive thirst, confusion and drowsiness. There was no history of cough, expectoration, chest pain, palpitation, headaches or visual disturbance. He had enjoyed good health and was not taking any drugs. There was no family history of diabetes or hypertension. He was a non-smoker but took 4–6 pints of lager over most weekends.

On examination he was dehydrated, disorientated and drowsy. Blood pressure was 90/60. Pulse was 112/min regular. Respiratory rate was 24/min. Temperature was 37°C. There was no anaemia, cyanosis, jaundice, oedema or clubbing. Thyroid and lymph nodes were not enlarged. Peripheral pulses were palpable except in the right dorsalis pedis artery. Examination of respiratory system, cardiovascular system and abdomen was normal. There was no neck stiffness, his fundi and cranial nerves were normal and there were no localizing neurological signs.

The following were the results of various initial investigations:

Haemoglobin 17.2 g/dl
WBC 11.0 × 10^9/l
MCV 83 fl
Sodium 149 mmol/l
Potassium 5.1 mmol/l
Chloride 100 mmol/l
Bicarbonate 22 mmol/l
Blood glucose (random) 47 mmol/l
Blood urea 15 mmol/l
Urine analysis – Glucose ++++; no ketones; protein trace
Chest X-ray normal
ECG – Sinus tachycardia; no infarct or ischaemic changes

Questions

1 What is the most likely diagnosis?
2 Give three important steps in the management of this patient.
3 What is the serum osmolality of this patient?

Answers to case 79

1 The most likely diagnosis in this 68-year-old gentleman with polyuria, polydipsia, confusion, drowsiness, dehydration, low blood pressure, rapid pulse and respiration, no neck stiffness, haemoconcentration (haemoglobin 17.2 g/dl), high serum sodium, hyperglycaemia and glycosuria with no ketonuria is hyperosmolar non-ketotic precoma. A previous history of diabetes may or may not be present in these patients.

2 (a) Volume replacement by half-strength saline
(b) Low-dose insulin therapy
(c) Correction of electrolyte imbalance

3 Serum osmolality may be calculated as

$$\text{Sodium} \times 2 + \text{Blood glucose} + \frac{\text{Urea}}{3}$$

$$149 \times 2 + 47 + \frac{15}{3} = 340 \text{ mOsmol}$$

CASE 80

A 43-year-old lady was rushed to the casualty department at about 9 pm with a history of drug (tricyclic antidepressant) overdose. She was divorced 2 months ago and had been depressed since then. Two weeks ago she was started on amytryptiline 25 mg three times a day by her doctor. It was estimated that she probably took 40–50 tablets altogether. She was seen about 5 pm by a neighbour, who found her collapsed near her bed at about 8 pm.

On examination she was unconscious and responded only to painful stimuli. Pulse was 116/min with frequent ectopics. Blood pressure was 110/60. Respiration was 18/min. JVP was not raised and there were no signs of clubbing or oedema. There were no heart murmurs but the tachycardia and frequent ectopics were confirmed on auscultation. Examination of respiratory system and abdomen proved normal. Her pupils were dilated but reacted normally to light. Conjunctival and corneal reflexes were normal. Fundi were normal. Deep reflexes were sluggish with normal plantar responses bilaterally.

Results of initial investigations were as follows:

Haemoglobin 13.9 g/dl
MCV 81 fl
WBC 8 × 10^9/l
Urea 10.4 mmol/l
Sodium 136 mmol/l
Potassium 4.1 mmol/l
Chloride 98 mmol/l
Creatinine 89 μmol/l
Chest X-ray – Normal lung fields. No cardiomegaly
Blood for drug screening – No salicylate or barbiturate detected

Questions

1 What are the cardiovascular complications of overdose with tricyclic antidepressants?
2 Give five contraindications of tricyclic antidepressant therapy.
3 Give four important steps for management of patients with tricyclic antidepressant overdose.

Answers to case 80

1 Cardiovascular side-effects are:
(a) Hypotension
(b) Tachycardia
(c) Heart blocks
(d) Cardiac asystole

2 The contraindications are:
(a) Recent myocardial infarction
(b) Heart blocks
(c) Patients on antihypertensive therapy, especially on bethanidine, clonidine, debrisoquine and guanethidine
(d) Glaucoma
(e) Hyperthyroidism

3 (a) Gastric lavage (activated charcoal may be helpful)
(b) Intravenous physostigmine 1–3 mg in cases of life-threatening arrhythmia, convulsion or coma
(c) Maintenance of airways
(d) Management of circulatory shock and metabolic acidosis

CASE 81

A 62-year-old lady was referred to the medical outpatient department for assessment of her leg oedema, painful knees and glycosuria. She had moved to a coastal resort with her husband who retired recently, and her new doctor was still waiting for her past medical record. She denied any history of chest pain, palpitation, cough or expectoration but had noticed that she was passing too much urine and hence the visit to the general practitioner. She had not been taking any drugs apart from occasional paracetamol. It transpired that the legs had been oedematous for at least 40 years, and her sister who died 4 years ago had a similar problem.

On examination she was obese, mentally alert and cheerful. JVP was not raised. She had bilateral non-pitting oedema of her legs. Blood pressure 140/70, pulse 80/min regular. There was no clubbing, jaundice, thyroid or lymph node enlargement. She was in sinus rhythm with no heart murmur. Respiratory and nervous system examination proved normal. Apart from osteoarthritis of both knees, other joints were clinically normal with good range of movements.

The following were the results of various investigations:

Haemoglobin 14.1 g/dl
ESR 21 mm/1st hour
Urea 10 mmol/l
Blood glucose 14.9 mmol/l
Urea and electrolytes normal
WBC 8 × 10^9/l
Urine analysis – Sugar ++; no albumin
Chest X-ray normal
ECG normal

Questions

1 What is the most likely diagnosis?
2 What is the mode of transmission of Milroy's disease?
3 Give three causes of secondary lymphoedema.

Answers to case 81

1 The most likely diagnosis in this 62-year-old lady with long-standing non-pitting (lymphatic) oedema of both legs, family history of similar disorder with no evidence of heart failure is Milroy's disease. The aetiology is probably congenital malformation of lymphatic channels. Besides Milroy's disease she has late-onset diabetes and osteoarthritis of knees.

2 The mode of inheritence is thought to be autosomal dominant.

3 (a) Invasion of lymph nodes by carcinomatosis
(b) Surgical removal of lymph nodes, e.g. in radical mastectomy
(c) Recurrent lymphangitis, e.g. filariasis common in tropics

CASE 82

Mrs A.J., a 72-year-old lady, was sent in by her general practitioner for assessment of confusion which she had for the past 6 months. Along with the confusion and odd behaviour she had been getting somewhat unsteady on her legs and had had at least two falls in the previous 4 weeks. She complained of a painful burning sensation in both legs. There was no history of cough, expectoration, chest pain, palpitation, urinary or bowel symptoms. She did not smoke or drink and had no significant previous illnesses.

On examination she was anaemic. Blood pressure was 160/100. Pulse was 78/min regular. Thyroid and lymph nodes were not enlarged. There was no clubbing, lymphadenopathy, or jaundice and her peripheral pulses were normal. She had a soft systolic murmur localized to the apex. Examination of respiratory system and abdomen proved normal. She was moderately confused. Cranial nerves were normal. There was loss of vibration sensation in both legs. Biceps, supinators and knee jerks were normal, but ankle jerks were absent on both sides. Plantar response was equivocal on the left side but the right plantar was upgoing.

The following were the results of various initial investigations:

Haemoglobin 9.8 g/dl
MCV 116 fl
ESR 30 mm/h
Sodium 137 mmol/l
Potassium 3.8 mmol/l
Chloride 100 mmol/l
Bicarbonate 24 mmol/l
Blood glucose 6.3 mmol/l
Blood urea 8.8 mmol/l
Chest X-ray normal
ECG normal

Questions

1 What is the most likely diagnosis?
2 What three further investigations will you ask for?
3 What other vitamin deficiencies may lead to dementia?
4 Give five causes of acute confusional state commonly seen in the elderly patients?

Answers to case 82

1 The most likely diagnosis in this elderly lady with a 6-month history of confusion, unsteadiness of legs, painful burning sensation in both legs, anaemia, loss of vibration sensation, absent ankle jerks, unequivocal left plantar and upgoing right plantar, low haemoglobin and high MCV is pernicious anaemia.

2 (a) Serum B_{12} and folate estimation
(b) Bone marrow examination
(c) Serological test for syphilis

3 B_1 and B_6 deficiencies.

4 (a) ***Infection – chest and urinary infections***

(b) ***Cardiovascular conditions such as myocardial infarction, heart failure and cardiac arrhythmias***

(c) ***Drug therapy such as anti-Parkinsonian drugs, antidepressants, hypnotics and sedatives***

(d) ***Metabolic conditions – dehydration, liver failure, kidney failure, thyroid disorders and electrolyte imbalance***

(e) ***Environmental changes such as a sudden change in the patient's environment, as seen on hospitalization.***

CASE 83

A 39-year-old lady was admitted with a 6-hour history of severe left-sided chest pain. For the past 4 months she had experienced increasing shortness of breath, and fatigue on exertion with swelling of her ankles. During the past 4 hours of her chest pain her breathlessness had worsened. There was no history of haemoptysis. She had mild unproductive cough for the past 3 months. The chest pain was described as sharp with no radiation, and was worse on deep breathing. She had been given frusemide 40 mg daily for her swollen legs and had also been started on digoxin 0.25 mg daily a week before her admission, arranged by her doctor. Her doctor had given her pethidine 50 mg parenterally before sending her to the hospital, but this had failed to control her pain. She had no known drug allergies. She lived with her husband in a ground-floor flat, had no children, had smoked 10 cigarettes a day for the past 20 years and enjoyed an occasional drink. She could remember having frequent sore throats as a child but there was no clear history of joint pains. One of her three brothers, however, had a heart condition and had been treated with aspirin and antibiotics for a long time.

On examination she was dyspnoeic and had mild central cyanosis. JVP was raised by 4 cm. There was moderate pitting oedema over both legs. Her throat was normal. Blood pressure was 120/70. Pulse was 108/min and irregular. There was no clubbing, thyroid or lymph node enlargement. Peripheral pulses were normal. Apex beat was tapping in character and she had a left parasternal heave. She was fibrillating at about 120/min at the apex. The first heart sound was loud and she had a rough, rumbling, mid-diastolic murmur localized to the apex. Opening snap followed closely on the second heart sound. She had bilateral basal crepitations with dullness and diminished air entry on her left base.

There was no pleural rub. Liver was 4 cm enlarged, smooth and tender. There was no splenomegaly or ascites. Fundi were normal and there were no localizing neurological signs.

The following results of the initial investigations were available:

Haemoglobin 12.8 g/dl
MCV 82 fl
Urea 9.8 mmol/l
Sodium 134 mmol/l
Potassium 3.6 mmol/l
Chloride 99 mmol/l
Bicarbonate 24 mmol/l
Blood glucose (random) 6 mmol/l
ECG – Confirmed atrial fibrillation; there were no ischaemic changes
Urine analysis — Protein trace; no sugar

Questions

1 What is the most likely diagnosis?
2 What four further investigations will help your diagnosis?
3 Give six important steps in the management of this patient.

Answers to case 83

1 ***The most likely diagnosis in this young lady with a 4-month history of increasing fatigue, shortness of breath, swelling of ankles with previous history of repeated sore throats and a family history of what appears to be rheumatic heart disease, with characteristic findings of mitral stenosis is rheumatic heart disease, mitral stenosis, atrial fibrillation and congestive cardiac failure. Sudden sharp pleuritic chest pain in a lady with mitral stenosis and atrial fibrillation strongly supports the diagnosis of pulmonary embolism. Systemic or pulmonary embolism is a common complication of mitral stenosis and may sometime be seen even in those patients who consistently remain in sinus rhythm. A pleuritic rub is not always present and may sometime be difficult to detect in the presence of diffuse crepitations.***

2 ***(a) Chest X-ray***
(b) Lung scan
(c) Pulmonary angiography
(d) Echocardiography

3 ***(a) Oxygen inhalation***
(b) Anticoagulation (start with heparin)
(c) Control of pain (morphine)
(d) Digoxin
(e) Diuretics, preferably given parenterally
(f) Consider using thrombolytic therapy (antistreptokinase)

CASE 84

A 76-year-old lady was admitted with a 3-month history of frequent falls. During the week preceding her admission she had two falls. The falls occurred without any prior warning and were not associated with loss of consciousness. She denied having any chest pain, but did admit to palpitation and giddiness lasting for a minute or so before the falls. She had previously been fit, and had not been taking any drugs.

On examination she was mentally alert. Blood pressure 140/80 sitting, 135/70 standing. There was no anaemia, clubbing or tremor. JVP was not raised. Examination of the joints was normal; in particular her neck movements were full without any associated giddiness. There were no carotid bruits. She was in sinus rhythm and had no heart murmur. Examination of respiratory and neurological systems proved normal.

The following were the results of various investigations:

Haemoglobin 13 g/dl
WBC 8 × 10^9/l
ESR 29 mm/h
Urea 6.7 mmol/l
Sodium 140 mmol/l
Potassium 3.4 mmol/l
Chloride 102 mmol/l
Bicarbonate 28 mmol/l
Total protein 62 g/l
Albumin 33 g/l
Bilirubin 12 μmol/l
Chest X-ray – Unfolding of the aorta; no cardiomegaly; lung fields are clear
ECG – Anterolateral ischaemic changes with occasional supraventricular and ventricular ectopics. A 24-h ECG recording helped to establish the diagnosis by showing brief runs of tachycardia and bradycardia associated with giddiness she had experienced before previous falls.

Questions

1 Give five cardiovascular causes of falls in the elderly.
2 How would you manage the patient described in the history?
3 What is a drop attack?

Answers to case 84

1 (a) Postural hypotension
(b) Cardiac arrhythmias (heart blocks, bradycardia, tachycardia)
(c) Transient ischaemic attacks (vertebrobasilar insufficiency)
(d) Aortic stenosis
(e) Myocardial infarction

2 This patient probably has a sick sinus syndrome causing tachybradycardia. A permanent pacemaker is indicated in such a situation.

3 Drop attacks are characterized by sudden falls without any warning or loss of consciousness. For some unknown reason drop attacks are almost always seen in middle-aged or elderly women. Falls occur only on walking rather than standing, and they often happen in the street and not indoors. The aetiology of drop attacks is far from being clear. In some patients at least they are thought to be associated with vertebrobasilar insufficiency.

CASE 85

A 37-year-old lady was sent to the outpatient department with a 5-month history of painful nodules on her legs, fatigue and tiredness. There was no history of cough, expectoration, chest pain, dyspnoea, palpitation, headaches, urinary or bowel symptoms. She had been taking the contraceptive pill for the past 8 years. She had smoked 20 cigarettes a day for the past 20 years but did not drink. She was married and had two children aged 13 and 10. There was no history of rheumatic heart disease, diabetes or hypertension.

On examination she was comfortable. She had no anaemia, jaundice, cyanosis or clubbing. Blood pressure was 130/70. Pulse was 74/min regular. Her throat was normal. JVP was not raised and her thyroid and lymph nodes were not enlarged. She had multiple nodular, tender lesions 2–4 cm in diameter on the anterior surface of both her legs. Examination of joints, cardiovascular and respiratory systems, abdomen and central nervous system proved unremarkable.

The following were the results of various initial investigations:

Haemoglobin 13.4 g/dl
ESR 24 mm/h
WBC 8.5 × 10^9/l
Sodium 139 mmol/l
Potassium 4.2 mmol/l
Chloride 100 mmol/l
Bicarbonate 23 mmol/l
Blood urea 4.9 mmol/l
Random blood glucose 5.8 mmol/l
ECG normal

Questions

1 What is the most likely diagnosis?
2 Give five causes of erythema nodosum.
3 What three further investigations would you ask for?

Answers to case 85

1 The most likely diagnosis in this 37-year-old lady with bilateral painful nodular lesions on her shin with no other abnormalities is erythema nodosum. Intake of oral contraceptives may or may not be related to erythema nodosum in this patient.

2 (a) Streptococcal infection
(b) Sarcoidosis
(c) Drug sensitivity (sulphonamides, oral contraceptives, aspirin, etc.)
(d) Tuberculosis
(e) Rheumatic fever

3 (a) Chest X-ray
(b) ASO (antistreptolysin O) titre
(c) Mantoux test

CASE 86

A man of 78, a known epileptic, was admitted with bone pains and difficulty in climbing stairs for the past 2 months. His appetite was normal and he had not lost any weight recently. There was no history of cough, chest pain or palpitation. He had had a tendency towards constipation for many years but had only recently been started on Senokot tablets by his own doctor. His epilepsy had been well controlled with phenytoin 100 mg in the morning and 200 mg at night, which he had been taking for the past year. He lived alone and was practically housebound, being visited by home help and neighbours regularly.

On examination he was mentally alert. He looked pale and had marked kyphoscoliosis but there was no clubbing, thyroid or lymph node enlargement. He had to be helped in getting out of the chair by two nurses, and could walk only a step or two. Cardiovascular and respiratory systems were normal. He had some evidence of proximal muscle wasting in his thighs but the tone and reflexes were normal.

Haemoglobin was reported as 9.8 g/dl with an MCV of 99. Results of other investigations were as follows:

ESR 40 mm/h
Total protein 64 g/l
Albumin 34 g/l
Bilirubin 17 μmol/l
Sodium 139 mmol/l
Potassium 3.7 mmol/l
Chloride 100 mmol/l
Bicarbonate 26 mmol/l
Blood urea 9.9 mmol/l
Blood glucose 7.2 mmol/l
ALT 30 u/l
Alkaline phosphatase 264 u/l

Questions

1 What is the most likely diagnosis, and why?
2 What else could be contributing to osteomalacia in this patient?
3 What is the cause of his anaemia?
4 What other four investigations would you ask for in this patient?

Answers to case 86

1 The most likely diagnosis in this elderly patient is osteomalacia. Induction of liver enzyme resulting in excessive metabolism of 25-hydroxycholecalciferol is not uncommon in patients taking phenytoin for a prolonged period.

2 In a housebound elderly patient lack of exposure to sunlight and inadequate intake of vitamin D, associated with poor nutrition, are other significant factors.

3 Macrocytic anaemia is one of the many side-effects of phenytoin therapy. Poor nutritional status (low folate intake) may also be contributing towards his anaemia.

4 (a) Serum calcium and phosphorus
(b) X-ray of bones (scapulae and pelvis) to look for pseudofractures
(c) Serum vitamin D level
(d) Serum B_{12} and folate levels

CASE 87

A 62-year-old lady was admitted with a 2-month history of progressive shortness of breath, tiredness and fatigue. In the week before her admission she had noticed some blood in her motions at least on four occasions but she had no abdominal pain, diarrhoea or sickness. There was no history of cough, expectoration or chest pain but she admitted having palpitation on moderate exertion. She was a non-smoker and did not take any alcohol. There was no history of previous significant illnesses.

On examination she was anaemic. Blood pressure was 130/70. Pulse was 88/min regular. JVP was normal. There was no clubbing, cyanosis, oedema, jaundice, thyroid or lymph node enlargement. There were a few telangiectasic lesions on her lips and oral mucosa. Her skin was otherwise normal. Examination of cardiovascular, respiratory and central nervous systems proved unremarkable. Her abdomen was soft and there was no hepatosplenomegaly. Rectal examination and sigmoidoscopy were normal.

The following were the results of various initial investigations:

Haemoglobin 8.9 g/dl
WBC 8.2 × 10^9/l
MCV 67 fl
Sodium 139 mmol/l
Potassium 3.4 mmol/l
Chloride 98 mmol/l
Bicarbonate 24 mmol/l
Blood urea 8.2 mmol/l
Random blood glucose 6.9 mmol/l
Chest X-ray normal
Barium enema normal

Questions

1 What is the most likely diagnosis?
2 What is the inheritance of hereditary haemorrhagic telangiectasia?
3 Give two measures commonly employed to treat patients with this condition.

Answers to case 87

1 The most likely diagnosis in this lady with history of progressive shorntess of breath, tiredness, fatigue, palpitation, rectal bleeding, anaemia with telangiectasic lesions on her lips and oral mucosa, low haemoglobin with low MCV, normal sigmoidoscopy and barium enema is hereditary haemorrhagic telangiectasia (Osler–Rendu–Weber syndrome).

2 The inheritance of this disorder is autosomal dominant.

3 (a) Continuous iron therapy
(b) Blood transfusion

CASE 88

Mrs N.C., a 70-year-old lady, was admitted with urinary and faecal incontinence for 2 days. She had severe osteoarthritis mainly affecting her knees and left hip, and had taken paracetamol regularly for at least 3 years. For past 3 weeks she was started on DF118 since paracetamol was not enough to control her pain. Because of her increasing pain she had been getting depressed for the past 6 months and had become almost housebound.

On examination she looked depressed and was mildly confused. JVP was not raised. Blood pressure was 140/70, pulse was regular, thyroid and lymph nodes were not enlarged. There was no clubbing, oedema or jaundice. She had painful limitation of movements of both knees and left hip. Her abdomen was distended and soft masses could be palpated all along the descending colon. The rectum was impacted with soft faeces.

Examination of cardiovascular and respiratory systems proved normal. There were no localizing neurological signs.

The following results were available:

Haemoglobin 13 g/dl
ESR 28 mm/1st hour
Total protein 65 g/l
Albumin 32 g/l
Sodium 142 mmol/l
Potassium 3.3 mmol/l
Chloride 98 mmol/l
Bicarbonate 25 mmol/l
WBC 6.7 × 10^9/l
Blood glucose 8.2 mmol/l
Blood urea 12 mmol/l

Her faecal impaction was treated with regular enemas and laxative and she was no more incontinent. She was sent home after 3 weeks of physiotherapy and rehabilitation.

Questions

1 What factors are responsible for this patient's faecal impaction?
2 Name four other drugs which commonly cause constipation in the elderly.
3 Give five complications of constipation.
4 What is the cause of urinary incontinence in this patient?

Answers to case 88

1 This patient has had poor mobility due to her arthritis and was started on DF118 (paracetamol and dihydrocodeine). Dihydrodeine is a morphine derivative and is well recognized to cause constipation. Further depression is a recognized cause of constipation leading to faecal impaction.

2 (a) Oral iron therapy
(b) Antidepressants – tricyclic group
(c) Anti-Parkinsonian drugs
(d) Diuretics causing dehydration

3 (a) Irritability and confusional state
(b) Faecal incontinence
(c) Obstruction
(d) Stercoral ulceration
(e) Megacolon

4 Pressure of a loaded rectum on the urethra and bladder interferes with the local reflexes and commonly causes urinary retention or incontinence in the elderly.

CASE 89

A 35-year-old bus driver presented to his doctor with a 3-week history of itchy rashes around his hands and fingers. His itching was worse at night and he had difficulty in sleeping at times. He enjoyed good health and had not taken any sick leave in the past 8 years since he had started his present job. He smoked 20 cigarettes a day and enjoyed occasional drinks. Six months ago he had gone to Spain on a 2-week holiday with his wife and two young children, aged 8 and 6. His wife and one son had also been complaining of itching all over for the past 5 days.

On examination he appeared fit and healthy. JVP was normal. Blood pressure was 150/90. Pulse was 80/min regular. There was no anaemia, cyanosis, jaundice, clubbing or oedema. Lymph nodes were not enlarged. On his hands he had fine, dark lines of scratching and eczematoid papular rashes in the finger webs. The rest of his skin and systemic examination was normal.

Results of the following investigations were available:

Haemoglobin 14.2 g/dl
White cell count 4.9×10^9/l
MCV 93 fl
Urea 7.1 mmol/l
Blood glucose 6.3 mmol/l
Sodium 137 mmol/l
Potassium 3.5 mmol/l
Bicarbonate 25 mmol/l
Chloride 96 mmol/l
Chest X-ray normal
Urine analysis – No protein or sugar

Questions

1 What is the most likely diagnosis?
2 How would you confirm the diagnosis?
3 Name two drugs which may be used to treat scabies.

Answers to case 89

1 The most likely diagnosis in this young patient with pruritic lesions on his hands and fingers, spreading to his family members, is scabies. Scabies is probably the most common skin condition associated with poor living conditions. It may sometimes be difficult to diagnose because scratching and secondary infection make the characteristic burrows in the finger webs difficult to recognize. The parasite causing scabies is the mite Sarcoptes scabiei.

2 Examination of skin scrapings using 10 per cent potassium hydroxide to demonstrate the parasite is a reliable method of establishing the diagnosis. The mite itself, or the eggs, may be seen in the film.

3 (a) Gamma benzene hexachloride (1 per cent cream)
(b) Benzyl benzoate (25 per cent emulsion)
It is important to remember that all members of the household should be treated simultaneously. Improvement in general living conditions and personal hygiene are also important in the prevention of reinfection.

CASE 90

A 74-year-old lady, a retired schoolteacher, was referred to the clinic with a 2-month history of generalized aches and pains and occasional headaches since the death of her husband. Her symptoms were only partially relieved by paracetamol tablets, six to eight tablets a day. In the past 3 weeks these pains worsened, she stopped going to the nearby day centre and had been feeling rather lonely and depressed. There was no history of cough, expectoration, chest pain or palpitation. She had lost about half a stone in weight in the past 2 months.

On examination she looked tired and pale. JVP was normal and there was no clubbing, lymphadenopathy or thyroid enlargement. Blood pressure was 160/90, pulse 78/min regular. She was noted to have some bruising over her right temporal region with localized hair loss and tender non-pulsatile temporal artery. Examination of the cardiovascular system and abdomen proved normal. All the cranial nerves were intact and the fundi were also normal. Motor, sensory system and reflexes, both superficial and deep, were present.

Routine investigations including haemoglobin, ESR, chest X-ray, liver function tests and urea and electrolytes were requested, and she was asked to attend again after a week for review with the results of all the investigations.

Her haemoglobin was reported as 10.6 g/dl and the ESR was found to be 46 mm/1st hour. Two days before she was due to attend for her next clinic appointment she woke up with moderately severe headache and difficulty in seeing things.

Results of the other investigations were as follows:

Blood urea 8.9 mmol/l
Sodium 137 mmol/l
Potassium 4.1 mmol/l
Chloride 99 mmol/l
Bicarbonate 24 mmol/l
Blood glucose 6.8 mmol/l
WBC 8×10^9/l
Urine analysis normal
Chest X-ray – Heart size normal; lung fields clear

Questions

1 What is the most likely diagnosis?
2 What course of action would you have taken had you seen her on her first visit?
3 Is the finding of an ESR of 46 mm/h inconsistent with the diagnosis?
4 How often is the temporal biopsy diagnostic?
5 How do you treat such patients?

Answers to case 90

1 The most likely diagnosis in this elderly lady presenting with aches and pains, depression, anaemia and tenderness over her right temporal region is temporal arteritis.

2 Instead of waiting to see her again after a week she should have had an urgent temporal artery biopsy and been started on high-dose steroids on the basis of strong suspicion of temporal arteritis.

3 ***No. Although in most cases the ESR is above 80 mm/h, this is not invariably the case. An ESR of 46 mm/h by no means rules out the diagnosis. At the same time it is important to remember that in many elderly an ESR of 40–50 mm/h may not be associated with any significant disease process.***

4 ***Only in about one-third of patients with cranial (temporal) arteritis is the biopsy positive. The diagnosis and the treatment must therefore never be solely based on biopsy results.***

5 ***Patients with temporal arteritis should be treated with high-dose steroids (over 30 mg a day) with the dose being adjusted both according to the falling ESR and symptomatic relief. The total time this therapy is required is usually about 2–3 years.***

CASE 91

A man of 68 was referred to the medical outpatient department with a 4-month history of progressive headache. His headache was diffused and generalized with no radiation. There was no history of blurring of vision, photophobia or vomiting and he had otherwise remained in good general health. There was no history of cough, expectoration, chest pain or palpitation. There were no urinary or bowel symptoms. His appetite had remained well and he had not lost any weight. There was no significant history of previous illness but for the past 3 months he had noticed some difficulty in hearing.

On examination he was comfortable. His blood pressure was 150/90, pulse was 78/min regular, thyroid and lymph nodes were not enlarged. There was no anaemia, cyanosis, jaundice or oedema. His head appeared to be enlarged with an irregular surface of the skull. Examination of the cardiovascular and respiratory systems and abdomen proved normal. Both Weber and Rinnie's test were indicative of eighth-nerve deafness on the left side. Other cranial nerves, motor and sensory systems were normal.

The following are the results of various investigations:

Haemoglobin 14.3 g/dl
Urea 9 mmol/l
Sodium 140 mmol/l
Potassium 4.0 mmol/l
Chloride 101 mmol/l
Bicarbonate 27 mmol/l
Blood sugar 8.9 mmol/l
WBC 6.7 × 10^9/l
MCV 82 fl
Serum calcium 2.2 mmol/l
Alkaline phosphatase 469 u/l

Questions

1 What is the most likely diagnosis?
2 What are the complications of Paget's disease?
3 Name three drugs which may be used for the treatment of active Paget's disease.

Answers to case 91

1 The most likely diagnosis in this 68-year-old gentleman with headaches, hearing difficulty, enlarged skull with irregular surface, evidence of nerve deafness and high serum alkaline phosphatase with normal serum calcium and phosphorus is Paget's disease of the bone.

2 (a) Bone pains
(b) Pathological fractures
(c) Cranial nerve palsy, most commonly of eighth nerve
(d) Congestive cardiac failure
(e) Osteogenic sarcoma

3 (a) Calcitonin
(b) Diphosphonates
(c) Mithramycin

CASE 92 A 36-year-old Irish woman was seen in the medical outpatient department with a 6-week history of progressive shortness of breath, tiredness and weight loss. Her appetite had been poor and she had lost 8 pounds in weight over the past 6 weeks. She had started with an unproductive cough which she thought was related to her smoking habits. There was no history of chest pain, palpitation, pruritus, night sweats, urinary or bowel symptoms. She denied having headaches or blurring of vision. She smoked 15 cigarettes a day but did not drink.

On examination she was comfortable. Her JVP was not raised and she had no oedema, clubbing, cyanosis or anaemia. Blood pressure was 130/80 mm, pulse 74/min and regular. Enlarged lymph nodes were palpable in both axillae, groins and supraclavicular regions. Thyroid was not palpable. Examination of cardiovascular system and abdomen proved normal. Trachea was central, chest expansion and auscultation was normal with normal vesicular breathing and no added sounds. Cranial nerves, motor and sensory system and reflexes were normal.

The following were the results of various investigations:

Haemoglobin 14.4 g/dl
ESR 23 mm/h
Blood urea 6.8 mmol/l
Blood glucose (random) 6.7 mmol/l
Sodium 137 mmol/l
Potassium 4.2 mmol/l
Chloride 98 mmol/l
Bicarbonate 26 mmol/l
Urine analysis normal
WBC 7.8 × 10^9/l
MCV 84 fl
Total protein 68 g/l
Serum albumin 48 g/l
Serum globulin 20 g/l
ECG normal
Chest X-ray – Bilateral hilar lymphandenopathy; clear lung fields

Questions

1 What is the most likely diagnosis?
2 What three further investigations will you request?
3 Give five indications for steroid therapy in sarcoidosis.

Answers to case 92

1 The most likely diagnosis in this 36-year-old Irish woman with history of progressive lymphadenopathy and bilateral hilar lymphadenopathy on the chest X-ray is sarcoidosis. Sarcoidosis is far more commonly seen in Irish people living in the United Kingdom. Tuberculosis and Hodgkin's disease must always be differentiated from sarcoidosis.

2 (a) Lymph node biopsy
(b) Kveim-Siltzbach test
(c) Pulmonary function tests

3 (a) Ocular involvement
(b) Progressive dyspnoea
(c) Persistent hypercalcaemia/hypercalciuria
(d) Disfiguring skin lesions
(e) Neurological involvement

CASE 93

A 58-year-old Pakistani immigrant was referred to the hospital with an 8-week history of bone pains, easy fatiguability and poor mobility. His appetite had remained unchanged but he had lost 5 pounds in weight over the past 8 weeks. There was no history of cough, expectoration, palpitation, urinary or bowel symptoms. He had lived in England for the past 3 years and was awaiting the arrival of his wife from Pakistan. He smoked 10 cigarettes a day but did not drink or take any medication.

On examination he was comfortable. Blood pressure was 150/80, pulse 74/min regular, thyroid and lymph nodes were not enlarged. He had no anaemia, cyanosis, jaundice or oedema. Examination of the joints proved normal. He was walking with a stick and had a waddling gait. Examination of cardiovascular and respiratory systems and abdomen proved normal. He had wasting of the proximal muscles of both thighs and needed help in getting up from the chair. Sensory system and reflexes were normal.

The following were the results of various investigations:

Haemoglobin 14.6 g/dl
ESR 19 mm/1st hour
Sodium 142 mmol/l
Potassium 3.9 mmol/l
Chloride 100 mmol/l
Bicarbonate 24 mmol/l
Blood urea 6.8 mmol/l
Blood glucose (random) 4.3 mmol/l
Urine analysis normal
WBC 7.8 × 10^9/l
MCV 81 fl
Total protein 69 g/l
Albumin 42 g/l
Globulin 27 g/l
Serum calcium 1.99 mmol/l
Serum phosphorus 1.01 mmol/l
Serum alkaline phosphatase 382 u/l

Questions

1 What is the most likely diagnosis?
2 What three further investigations will help your diagnosis?
3 Give four other causes of proximal myopathy.

Answers to case 93

1 The most likely diagnosis in this Asian immigrant with history of bone pains, easy fatiguability, weight loss, normal joints with proximal muscle weakness and waddling gait with low serum calcium and high alkaline phosphatase is osteomalacia.

2 (a) Skeletal survey to look for Looser's zones
(b) Bone scan
(c) Bone biopsy

3 (a) Corticosteroid therapy
(b) Polymyalgia rheumatica
(c) Carcinomatosis
(d) Thyrotoxicosis

CASE 94

A 29-year-old housewife was seen in the medical outpatient department with a 4-week history of fever, fatigue and weight loss. Her temperature was noted to be irregular and only mildly elevated without any associated chills or rigors. She had poor appetite and had lost 8 pounds in weight over the past 4 weeks. There was no history of cough, expectoration, chest pain, palpitation or night sweats. She had no urinary or bowel symptoms. She was happily married and had an 8-year-old daughter. She smoked 10 cigarettes a day but did not drink. She had not been taking any medication. There was no history of rheumatic heart disease but her brother had been treated for a heart condition for the past 15 years.

On examination she was pale, blood pressure was 120/70 mm. Pulse was 88/min and regular. She had clubbing of her fingers but there was no cyanosis, thyroid or lymph node enlargement. JVP was not raised. She had petechial haemorrhages in her left conjunctiva. Heart was in sinus rhythm. First heart sound was loud and she had a mid-diastolic localized murmur at the apex. Splenic tip was easily palpable but she had no hepatomegaly or ascites. Examination of respiratory and central nervous systems proved normal.

The following were the results of various investigations:

Haemoglobin 10.2 g/dl
ESR 48 mm/1st hour
Sodium 135 mmol/l
Potassium 4.2 mmol/l
Chloride 96 mmol/l
Bicarbonate 23 mmol/l
Blood urea 4.9 mmol/l
Blood glucose (random) 8.1 mmol/l
WBC 8 × 10^9/l
MCV 83 fl
Total protein 62 g/l
Albumin 34 g/l
Globulin 28 g/l
Urine analysis – No glucose or ketones; 4–8 RBC/HPF

Questions

1 What is the most likely diagnosis?
2 What three further investigations will you ask for?
3 Name three complications of infective endocarditis.

Answers to case 94

1 The most likely diagnosis in this young lady with 4-week history of pyrexia, fatigue, weight loss, anaemia, clubbing, petechial haemorrhages with a characteristic murmur of mitral stenosis, splenomegaly, raised ESR and haematuria is infective endocarditis. Unexplained fever in a patient with a heart murmur should always arouse suspicion of endocarditis. A clear-cut history of rheumatic heart disease is available in only 50 per cent of patients. In fact, her brother had a rheumatic valvular lesion and attended for a regular checkup.

2 (a) Blood cultures
(b) Chest X-ray
(c) ECG

3 (a) Systemic or pulmonary embolization
(b) Cardiac failure
(c) Renal failure

CASE 95

A 42-year-old accountant was seen in the medical outpatient department with a 7-month history of excessive sweating, pain and stiffness of his fingers. His appetite had remained unchanged but he had gained 5 pounds in weight over the past 7 weeks. He admitted to having occasional headaches which settled on taking paracetamol. There was no history of cough, expectoration, chest pain or palpitation. He had no urinary or bowel symptoms. He was married and had a 9-year-old son. His marital relationship with his wife had been strained since he had been gradually losing his interest in sexual activities over the past 6 months. He did not smoke or drink.

He appeared to be a man of large frame. His lower jaw appeared to be protruding. Facial features were rather coarse with prominent lips, nose and ears. Blood pressure was 170/100, pulse 78/min regular, and his JVP was not raised. Thyroid and lymph nodes were not enlarged. There was no anemia, cyanosis, jaundice or oedema. His joints were not swollen. Examination of respiratory and cardiovascular systems and abdomen proved normal. Visual acuity was normal but his fundi showed grade 2 changes of hypertension. He was also found to have a visual field defect affecting his temporal regions on both sides. The rest of the cranial nerves, motor and sensory system and reflexes were normal.

The following were the results of various investigations:

Haemoglobin 13.9 g/dl
ESR 23 mm/h
Sodium 142 mmol/l
Potassium 4.1 mmol/l
Chloride 100 mmol/l
Bicarbonate 25 mmol/l
Blood sugar 13 mmol/l
Blood urea 10 mmol/l
WBC 8.7 $\times$ 10^9/l
MCV 80 fl
Chest X-ray – Moderate cardiomegaly; clear lung fields
Urine analysis – Glucose ++

Questions

1 What is the most likely diagnosis?
2 What three further investigations will you ask for?
3 Give two other modes of presentation of acromegaly.

Answers to case 95

1 The most likely diagnosis in this gentleman with history of excessive sweating, pain and stiffness of fingers (arthralgia), weight gain, headaches, loss of libido, coarse facial features with prognathism, hypertension with retinopathy and cardiomegaly, bitemporal visual field defect, hyperglycaemia and glucosuria, is acromegaly.

2 (a) X-ray of skull, hands and feet
(b) Estimation of serum growth hormone level
(c) ECG

3 (a) Paraesthesia of the hands and feet
(b) Change in size of the hat, ring or shoes

CASE 96 A 28-year-old schoolteacher was seen in the medical outpatient department with a 6-week history of swelling of the face, hands and legs. She was getting exessively worried about the puffiness of her face in the mornings. Swelling of the hands and legs was usually worse towards the evenings. Her appetite had not changed but she had gained 6 pounds over the past 6 weeks. There was no history of cough, sore throat, expectoration, chest pain, palpitation, urinary or bowel symptoms. She smoked 15 cigarettes a day and took alcohol occasionally. She was not on any medication apart from occasional paracetamol for her tension headaches. There was no significant history of previous illness.

On examination, her blood pressure was 120/80, pulse 78/min regular. JVP was not raised and she was not dysphoeic. She had mild periorbital puffiness but marked pitting oedema of both legs. There was no anaemia, cyanosis, jaundice, or clubbing. She did not have any spider naevi or Dupuytren's contractures. Examination of respiratory, cardiovascular and central nervous systems proved unremarkable. There was no ascites, hepatosplenomegaly or renal enlargement.

The following were the results of various investigations:

Haemoglobin 13.6 g/dl
ESR 22 mm/1st hour
Sodium 134 mmol/l
Potassium 3.6 mmol/l
Chloride 96 mmol/l
Bicarbonate 24 mmol/l
Blood Urea 7.8 mmol/l
Blood glucose (random) 4.9 mmol/l
WBC 8 × 10^9/l
MCV 87 fl
Total proteins 48 g/l
Total albumin 21 g/l
Total globulin 27 g/l
ECG normal
Chest X-ray – Heart size normal limits; lung fields clear
Urine analysis – Glucose absent; protein ++++; RBC/WBC – O; hyaline casts 4–6/HRF

Questions

1 What is the most likely diagnosis?
2 What four further investigations will help your diagnosis?
3 Give five important causes of nephrotic syndrome in adults.

Answers to case 96

1 The most likely diagnosis in this 28-year-old schoolteacher with history of swelling of face, hands and legs, weight gain (fluid retention), no evidence of liver cell disease (no spider naevi or Dupuytren's contracture), hypoproteinaemia and heavy proteinuria is nephrotic syndrome.

2 (a) Serum protein electrophoresis
(b) 24 h urinary protein estimation
(c) Antinuclear antibody (ANA) titre
(d) Renal biopsy

3 (a) *Glomerulonephritis*
(b) *Pyelonephritis*
(c) *Diabetes mellitus*
(d) *Collagen diseases, e.g. systemic lupus erythemotosus*
(e) *Amyloidosis*

CASE 97

A 48-year-old Indian gentleman was brought to the casualty department with a 2-day history of fever, chills, rigors and headaches. There was no history of cough, expectoration, chest pain, palpitation, urinary or bowel symptoms. He had no photophobia, blurring of vision or vomiting. His son, with whom he had come to stay 3 weeks ago from India, thought that his father had been getting confused for the past 6–8 hours.

On examination he was confused and disorientated. BP was 140/85, pulse 98/min regular. JVP was not raised and there was no anaemia, cyanosis, jaundice, oedema or clubbing. Temperature was 39°C, peripheral pulses were palpable. Examination of respiratory and cardiovascular systems and abdomen proved unremarkable. Motor and sensory system and reflexes were normal. There was no neck stiffness.

The following were the results of various investigations:

Haemoglobin 13.2 g/dl
Blood urea 7.9 mmol/l
Blood glucose (random) 8.4 mmol/l
Sodium 139 mmol/l
Potassium 4.2 mmol/l
Chloride 99 mmol/l
Bicarbonate 25 mmol/l
Urine analysis – Trace protein; no RBC/WBC; no glucose
WBC 8.9 × 10^9/l
MCV 79 fl
ECG Sinus tachycardia
Chest X-ray – Heart size normal; lung fields clear

Questions

1 What is the most likely diagnosis?
2 What single further investigation will you ask for?
3 How do you treat the acute attack of malaria?

Answers to case 97

1 The most likely diagnosis in this Indian gentleman with a history of fever with chills and rigors, headaches with no neck stiffness, acute confusional state, no localizing neurological signs with no signs of acute phelonephritis (no renal tenderness) is malaria.

2 Confirmation of the diagnosis depends on demonstration of the parasite in the stained blood smear. More than one smear may be required at times.

3 Except for drug-resistant falciparum malaria, the drug of choice in all cases is chloroquine. The usual course consists of 1 g of chloroquine phosphate given as a stat. dose followed by 500 mg after 6 hours and then 500 mg daily for next 2 days. For chloroquine-resistant cases use of quinine or pyrimethamine is recommended.

CASE 98

A 58-year-old woman, a known hypertensive for the past 12 years, was admitted with a 3-month history of shortness of breath and palpitations on moderate exertion. She had no history of cough, expectoration or chest pain. Her appetite had remained unchanged but she had gained about 6 pounds in weight over the past 3 months. Her bowels were normal and she had no urinary symptoms. She did not smoke or drink. Her only medication was methyldopa, 500 mg three times a day, which she had been taking for the past 10 years for the control of her blood pressure.

On examination she was markedly anaemic. Blood pressure was 160/100, pulse 96/min, respiration was 20/min. Her JVP was raised by 3 cm. Thyroid and lymph nodes were not enlarged and she had no clubbing or cyanosis. Trachea was central, chest expansion was fair and equal on both sides. She had bilateral basal crepitations. Heart sounds were normal with no murmur. Examination of the abdomen and central nervous system proved normal.

Results of the various investigations were as follows:

Haemoglobin 8 g/dl
ESR 18 mm/h
Urea 8.3 mmol/l
Sodium 138 mmol/l
Potassium 3.5 mmol/l
Chloride 99 mmol/l
Bicarbonate 24 mmol/l
Total protein 69 g/l
Albumin 45 g/l
Globulin 24 g/l
WBC 6 × 10^9/l
MCV 89 fl
Reticulocytes 5%
Chest X-ray – Heart size enlarged with evidence of pulmonary congestion
ECG – Left ventricular hypertrophy

Questions

1 What is the most likely diagnosis?
2 Give three other conditions associated with autoimmune haemolytic anaemia.
3 Give three causes of reticulocytosis.

Answers to case 98

1 The most likely diagnosis in this patient with known hypertension on methyldopa therapy for over 10 years, dyspnoea and palpitation on exertion, anaemia, tachycardia, tachypnoea with bilateral basal crepitations, abnormal ECG and chest X-ray and reticulocytosis is hypertension, congestive cardiac failure and haemolytic anaemia, most probably related to methyldopa intake. Ten to twenty per cent of patients on prolonged methyldopa therapy develop a positive Coombs' test. Autoimmune haemolytic anaemia, however is seen in less than 2 per cent of these patients.

2 (a) Chronic lymphatic leukaemia
(b) Lymphoma
(c) Systemic lupus erythematosus

3 (a) Haemolytic anaemia
(b) Patients on therapy with iron, B_{12} or folic acid
(c) Haemorrhage

CASE 99

A 30-year-old office clerk was sent to the medical outpatient department with a 2-month history of polyuria and increased thirst. He passed large amounts of urine with daytime frequency of six to eight times, and had to wake up at least once in the night. There was no history of dysuria. He denied having any cough, expectoration, chest pain, palpitation or headaches. His bowels were normal and there was no history of loss of appetite or weight. He did not smoke or drink and was happily married. There was no significant history of past illnesses and he was not taking any drugs.

On examination he appeared to be fit. His blood pressure was 130/70, pulse 74/min regular, JVP not raised. He had no oedema, clubbing, thyroid or lymph node enlargement. Examination of the respiratory system, abdomen and cardiovascular system proved normal. His fundi were normal and there were no localizing neurological signs.

The following were the results of various investigations:

Haemoglobin 14.3 g/dl
ESR 23 mm/1st hour
Blood urea 4.9 mmol/l
Blood glucose 5.4 mmol/l
Sodium 138 mmol/l
Potassium 3.9 mmol/l
Chloride 102 mmol/l
Bicarbonate 25 mmol/l
Total proteins 70 g/dl
Albumin 45 g/dl
Globulin 25 g/dl
WBC 8 × 10^9/l
MCV 83 fl
Chest X-ray normal
ECG normal
Serum calcium 2.15 mmol/l
Serum phosphorus 0.9 mmol/l
Serum alkaline phosphatase 120 u/l
Urinary osmolality 190 mOsmol

Questions

1 What is the most likely diagnosis?
2 Give six causes of polyuria.
3 How do you differentiate diabetes insipidus (both pituitary and nephrogenic) from compulsive water-drinking?

Answers to case 99

1 The most likely diagnosis in this patient with polyuria with normal blood glucose, urea and electrolyte and serum calcium, a stable personality and low urinary osmolality is diabetes insipidus.

2 (a) Diabetes mellitus
(b) Diabetes insipidus
(c) Compulsive water-drinking
(d) Chronic renal failure
(e) Hypercalcaemia
(f) Hypokalaemia

3 The following table summarizes the three conditions.

	Diabetes insipidus (pituitary)	*Diabetes insipidus* (nephrogenic)	Compulsive water-drinking
Urine osmolality	***Low (less than 200 mOsmol)***	***Low***	***Low***
Plasma osmolality	***Normal/high (280–310 mOsmol)***	***Normal/high***	***Normal/Low***
Water deprivation test	***Urine osmolality remains low***	***Low urinary osmolality***	***Urine osmolality is significantly increased (more than 700 mOsmol)***
Pitressin test	***Urine osmolality significantly increased***	***Urine osmolality is unaffected***	***Urine osmolality is increased***
Plasma ADH	***Low***	***High***	***Low***

CASE 100

A 48-year-old headmaster was referred to the medical outpatient with a 6-week history of weight loss, anorexia, left flank pain and intermittent pyrexia. He had lost 8 pounds in weight over the past 6 weeks. He complained of constant dull aching pain in the left flank which was not related to intake of food, change of posture or defaecation. He had no history of cough, expectoration, chest pain, palpitation, urinary or bowel symptoms. He smoked 20 cigarettes a day but did not drink or take any medication. There was no history of significant past illnesses.

On examination he was thinly built and anaemic. Blood pressure was 125/80, pulse 78/min regular. There was no clubbing, cyanosis, jaundice, oedema, thyroid, or lymph node enlargement. Examination of cardiovascular, respiratory and central nervous system was normal. Abdomen was soft with an enlarged left kidney but there was no ascites or hepatosplenomegaly. Rectal examination was normal with no prostatic enlargement. Scrotal examination revealed a left-sided varicocele.

Results of various investigations were as follows:

Haemoglobin 11.2 g/dl
ESR 98 mm/1st hour
Blood urea 7.4 mmol/l
Blood glucose 4.9 mmol/l
Sodium 134 mmol/l
Potassium 3.8 mmol/l
Chloride 98 mmol/l
Bicarbonate 25 mmol/l
WBC 6×10^9/l
MCV 79 fl
ECG normal
Chest X-ray – Heart size within normal limits; lung fields clear
Urine analysis – No sugar; RBCS +++

Questions

1 What is the most likely diagnosis?
2 What further investigations will help your diagnosis?

Answers to case 100

1 The most likely diagnosis in this 48-year-old patient with history of weight loss, anorexia, left flank pain, pyrexia, anaemia, left renal enlargement, left-sided varicocele, haematuria and high ESR is hypernephroma. Renal carcinoma is an important cause of pyrexia of unknown origin and may sometimes be associated with hypertension, polycythaemia, leukemoid reaction, hypercalcaemia and amyloidosis.

2 (a) Abdominal ultrasound
(b) Abdominal CT scan
(c) Selective angiography

NORMAL LAB VALUES IN ADULTS

Haemoglobin — Males 13–18 g/dl; females 12–16 g/dl
RBC — Males 5–6.5 × 10^6/mm^3; females 4–5.5 × 10^6/mm^3
WBC 4000–11,000/mm^3
Neutrophils 50–70%
Lymphocytes 20–40%
Monocytes 2–10%
Eosinophils 0–4%
Basophils 0–1%
MCV 76–96 μm^3
MCH 27–32 $\mu\mu$g
MCHC 32–38%
Reticulocytes 0.5–2%
Platelets 150,000–500,000/mm^3
ESR
- Westergren — Males 3–5 mm; females 4–7/mm
- Wintrobe — Males 0–9/mm; females 0–20/mm

Sodium 136–145 mmol/l
Potassium 3.5–5.0 mmol/l
Chloride 95–105 mmol/l
Bicarbonate 22–28 mmol/l
Urea 2.5–7.5 mmol/l
Creatinine 60–130 μmol/l
Calcium 2.1–2.6 mmol/l
Phosphorus 0.8–1.4 mmol/l
Total protein 60–80 g/l
Albumin 30–50 g/l
Globulin 20–30 g/l
Total bilirubin 5–17 μmol/l
AST — Up to 25 u/l
ALT — Up to 20 u/l
Serum alkaline phosphatase 20–100 u/l
Serum amylase 80–160 Somogyi units/100ml
CPK — Up to 100 u/l
GGT — Up to 60 ul/male; up to 40 ul/female
T4 — Adults 55–14.4 nmol/l (40–110 μg/l)
T4-free — Adults 10–30 pmol/l (0.8–2.3 ng/100ml)
TBG — Adults 12–30 mg/l
TSH — Adults 1–5 miu/l
T3 — Adults 0.9–2.8 nmol/l (0.7–2 μg/1)
Vitamin D — Adults and children 10–80 nmol/1 (4–32 ng/ml)
Cholestrol 125–250 mg/dl
Triglycerides 50–200 mg/dl
Glucose 3.9–5.6 mmol/l
pO_2 10–13.3 kPa (75–100 mmHg)
pCO_2 4.7–6 kPa (35–45 mmHg)
Serum iron 12–26 μmol/l (66–145 μg/100 ml)
Serum iron binding capacity 45–70 μmol/l (250–400 μg/100 ml)
Serum ferritin — males 24–400 μg/l; Females 15–300 μg/l
Folate
- Serum 3–16 μg/l (3–16 ng/ml)
- Red cell 200–600 ng/1 (200–600 pg/ml)

Serum vitamin B_{12} 150–900 ng/l (150–900 pg/ml)

INDEX OF CASE STUDIES

(This index lists the case study numbers.)